The Anti-Inflammatory Diet Soups and Stews Cookbook

Discover the Anti-Inflammatory Power of
Delicious, Simple, and Natural
Soups and Stews

By
Olga Jones

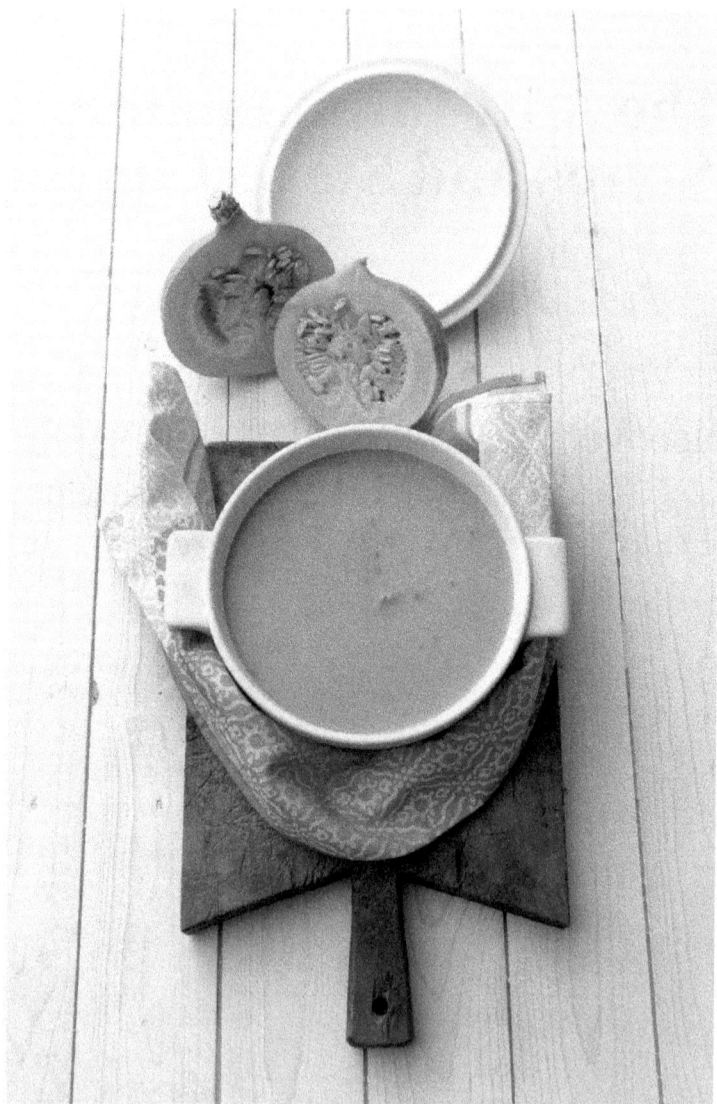

the publisher or the original author of this work can be in any fashion deemed liable for any hardship or damages that may befall them after undertaking information described herein.

Additionally, the information in the following pages is intended only for informational purposes and should thus be thought of as universal. As befitting its nature, it is presented without assurance regarding its prolonged validity or interim quality. Trademarks that are mentioned are done without written consent and can in no way be considered an endorsement from the trademark holder.

Table of Contents

INTRODUCTION

What is the Anti-Inflammatory Diet?

The anti-inflammatory diet is the best choice for your health if you have conditions that cause inflammation. Such conditions are asthma, chronic peptic ulcer, tuberculosis, rheumatoid arthritis, periodontitis, Crohn's disease, sinusitis, active hepatitis, etc. Along with medical treatment, proper nutrition is very important. An anti-inflammatory diet can help to reduce the pain from inflammation for a few notches. Such a diet isn't a panacea but a significant help in any treatment. Inflammation is a natural response of your body to infections, injuries, and illnesses. The classic symptoms of inflammation are redness, pain, heat, and swelling. Nevertheless, some diseases don't have any symptoms. Such illnesses are diabetes, heart disease, cancer, etc. That's why we should care about our health permanently and an anti-inflammatory diet is one of the ways for it.

Inflammation is your immune system's response to injury or unwanted microbes in your body. It is a natural process and vital part of your body's healing process. When inflammation becomes systemic and chronic, however, it becomes a problem, and measures need to be taken. This type of inflammation serves no purpose, and can cause a lot of harm to the body.

This book has a LOT of recipes, and not every recipe might work for you. For example, if you're allergic to dairy or gluten, the recipes containing those ingredients will cause more harm than good. However, substitutions are possible for all of these, so you will be fine following this book as long as you keep an eye on the ingredients and use a bit of creativity where you have to! Once you understand the fundamentals of the diet, you will be fully equipped to create your own recipes from scratch!This is the most important information that you should know before starting a diet. Any diet is not a magic remedy for all diseases; it is a support for the body during a difficult time of treatment. Start your new healthy life from one small step and you will see the huge results within half a year. You can be sure that your body will be thankful to you by giving you a fresh look and energy for new achievements.

Spring Pea Soup

Time To Prepare: five minutes
Time to Cook: fifteen minutes
Yield: Servings 6

Ingredients:
- ½ tsp. Black pepper powder
- ½ tsp. ground cumin
- 1 liter Vegetable stock
- 1 medium Chopped onion
- 2 tbsp. Coconut oil
- 2 tsp. Celtic sea salt
- 700 g. Fresh peas
- Chopped flat-leaf parsley
- Chopped mint leaves
- Fresh lemon juice
- Grated nutmeg
- Toasted sunflower seeds

Directions:
1. Warm the coconut oil in a pan set on moderate heat.
2. Mix in onions and stir fry for approximately five minutes.
3. Put in the stock and raise the heat.
4. Throw in fresh peas and cook for five minutes. If you're using frozen peas, it should take half the time.
5. Pour in the lemon juice, salt, pepper, herbs, and spices stirring continuously
6. Remove the heat and allow it to cool before running it through a food processor to whatever consistency you prefer.

7. Serve with sunflower seed sprinkles and mint or parsley leaves.

8. Enjoy!

Bacon & Cheese Soup

Time To Prepare: fifteen minutes
Time to Cook: forty minutes
Yield: Servings 6

Ingredients:
- ½ cup sour cream, for serving
- ½ teaspoon cumin
- ½ teaspoon onion powder
- ½ teaspoon paprika
- 1 cup heavy cream
- 1 cup shredded cheddar cheese
- 1 pound of lean ground beef
- 1 tablespoon coconut oil, for cooking
- 1 teaspoon garlic powder
- 1 yellow onion, chopped
- 6 cups beef broth
- 6 slices uncured bacon

Directions:
1. Put in the coconut oil to a frying pan and cook the bacon until crunchy.
2. Allow the bacon to cool and cut into little pieces. Set aside.
3. Once cooked, put in the lean ground beef to the same frying pan with the bacon fat and cook until browned.
4. Put in the onions and cook for an extra two to three minutes.
5. Put in all the ingredients minus the bacon, heavy cream, sour cream and cheese to a stock pot and stir.
6. Cook for about twenty-five minutes.

7. Warm the heavy cream, and then put in the warmed cream and cheese and serve with the bacon and a spoonful of sour cream

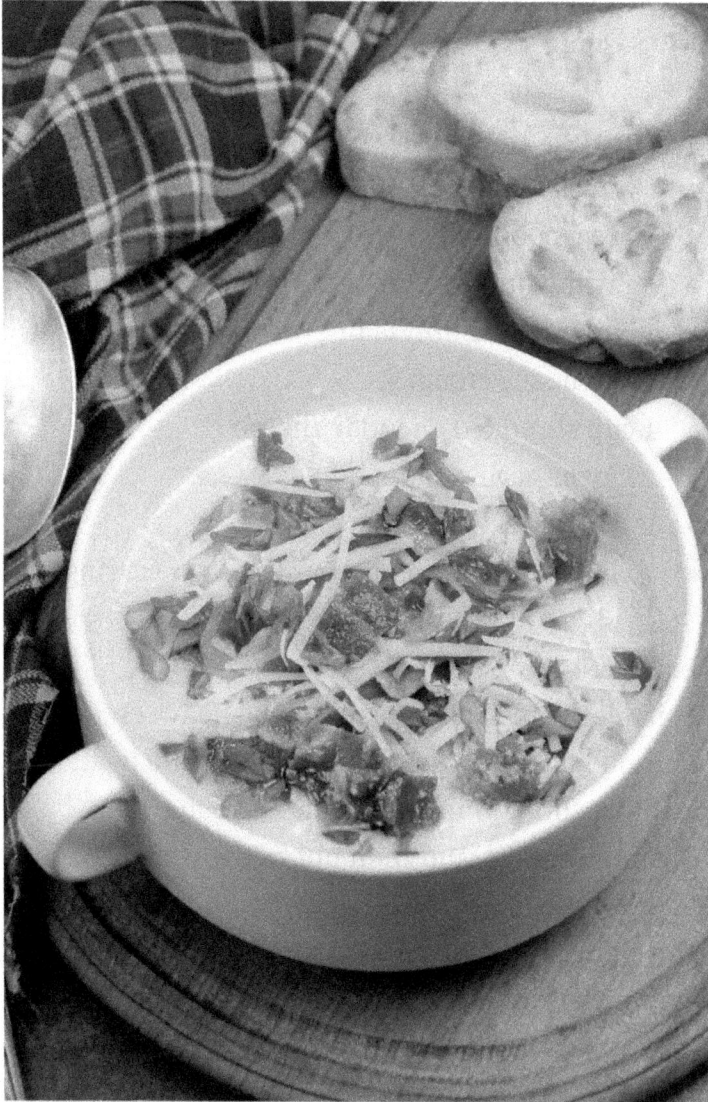

Broccoli Cheddar & Bacon Soup

Time To Prepare: ten minutes
Time to Cook: ten minutes
Yield: Servings 6

Ingredients:
- ¼ teaspoon black pepper
- ½ teaspoon salt
- ½ white onion, chopped
- 1 cup broccoli florets finely chopped
- 1 cup heavy cream
- 1 cup shredded cheddar cheese
- 2 cloves garlic, chopped
- 2 cups chicken broth
- 3 slices cooked bacon, crumbled for serving

Directions:
1. Put in all the ingredients minus the heavy cream, cheddar cheese and bacon to a stockpot on moderate heat.
2. Heat to a simmer and cook for 5 minutes.
3. Warm the cream, and then put in the warm cream and cheddar cheese.
4. Whisk until the desired smoothness is achieved.
5. Serve with crumbled bacon.

Brown Rice and Shitake Miso Soup with Scallion

Time To Prepare: ten minutes
Time to Cook: forty-five minutes
Yield: Servings 4

Ingredients:
- ½ teaspoon salt
- 1 (1½-inch) piece fresh ginger, peeled and cut
- 1 cup medium grain brown rice
- 1 cup thinly cut shiitake mushroom caps
- 1 garlic clove, minced
- 1 tablespoon white miso
- 2 scallions, thinly cut
- 2 tablespoons finely chopped fresh cilantro
- 2 tablespoons sesame oil

Directions:
1. In a large pot, heat the oil on moderate to high heat.
2. Put in the mushrooms, garlic, and ginger and sauté until the mushrooms start to tenderize, approximately five minutes.
3. Place the rice and stir to uniformly coat with the oil.
4. Put in 2 cups of water and salt and place it to its boiling point.
5. Reduce the heat then cook until the rice is soft, thirty to forty minutes.
6. Use a little of the soup broth to tenderize the miso, then mix it into the pot until well mixed. 7. Stir in the scallions and cilantro, then serve.

Butternut Squash Soup with Shrimp

Time To Prepare: ten minutes
Time to Cook: twenty minutes
Yield: Servings 4

Ingredients:

- ¼ cup slivered almonds (not necessary)
- ¼ teaspoon freshly ground black pepper
- 1 cup unsweetened almond milk
- 1 garlic clove, cut
- 1 pound cooked peeled shrimp, thawed if required
- 1 small red onion, finely chopped
- 1 teaspoon salt
- 1 teaspoon turmeric
- 2 cups peeled butternut squash cut into ¼-inch dice
- 2 tablespoons finely chopped fresh flat-leaf parsley
- 2 teaspoons grated or minced lemon zest
- 3 cups vegetable broth
- 3 tablespoons unsalted butter

Directions:

1. In a large pot, melt the butter on high heat.
2. Put in the onion, garlic, turmeric, salt, and pepper and sauté until the vegetables are tender and translucent, five to seven minutes.
3. Put in the broth and squash and bring to its boiling point.
4. Reduce the heat and cook until the squash has tenderized, approximately five minutes. Put in the shrimp and almond milk and cook until thoroughly heated, approximately 2 minutes.
5. Drizzle with the almonds (if using), parsley, and lemon zest before you serve

Carrot Broccoli Stew

Time To Prepare: ten minutes
Time to Cook: forty-five minutes
Yield: Servings 3

Ingredients:
- 1 cup Broccoli, florets
- 1 cup Carrots, cut
- 1 cup Heavy Cream
- 3 cups Chicken broth Salt and black pepper to taste

Directions:
1. Put in florets, cream, carrots, salt, and chicken broth; toss thoroughly.
2. Secure the lid and cook on Meat/Stew mode for forty minutes on High.
3. When ready, do a quick pressure release.
4. Move into serving bowls and drizzle black pepper on top

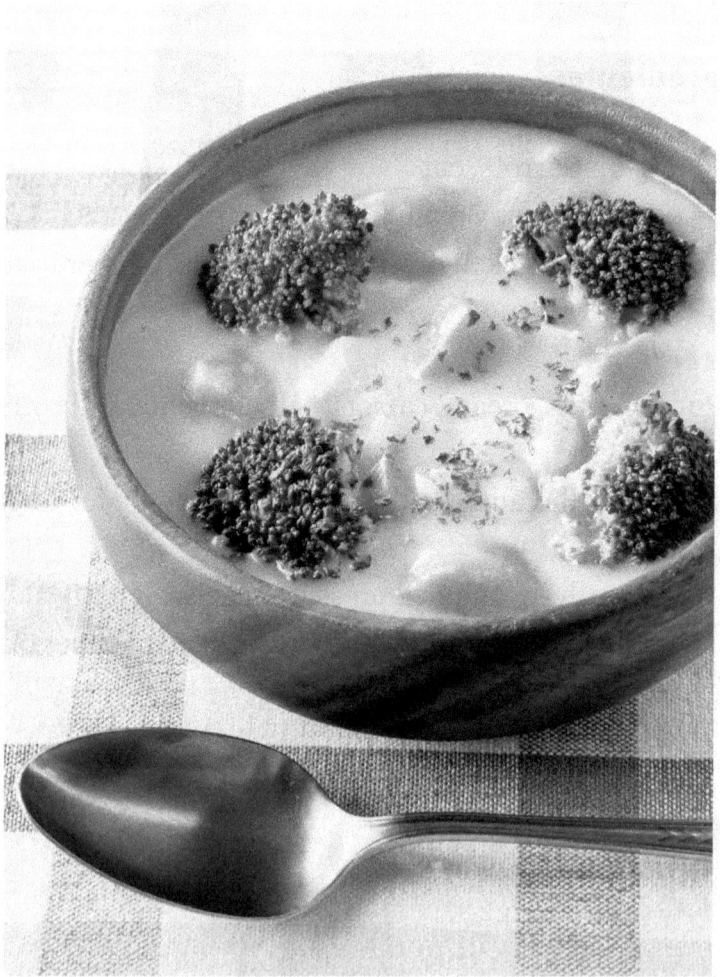

Cauliflower And Clam Chowder

Time To Prepare: ten minutes
Time to Cook: ten minutes
Yield: Servings 6

Ingredients:
- ½ teaspoon dried thyme
- 1 small yellow onion
- 1½ cups heavy whipping cream
- 3 (6.5-ounce / 184-g) cans chopped clams
- 3 tablespoons butter
- 4 cups chopped cauliflower

From the cupboard:
- Salt and freshly ground black pepper, to taste

Directions:
1. Split the clams and clam juice into two bowls.
2. Thin the clam juice with water to make 2 cups of juice.
3. Place the onion and butter in an instant pot and press the Sauté bottom, then sauté for a couple of minutes or until the onion is translucent.
4. Put in the clam juice and cauliflower into the instant pot.
5. Place the lid on and press the Manual button, and set the temperature to 375°F (190°C), then cook for five minutes.
6. Quick Release the pressure, then open the lid and mix in the heavy cream and clams.
7. Push the Sauté bottom and cook for about three minutes or until the clams are opaque and firm, then drizzle with thyme, salt, and black pepper.
8. Stir to mix thoroughly. Ladle the chowder in a big container and serve warm.

Celery Soup

Time To Prepare: ten minutes
Time to Cook: twenty minutes
Yield: Servings 4

Ingredients:
- ½ cup brown onion, chopped
- ½ cup full-fat milk
- ½ pound with Salsiccia links, casing removed and cut
- ½ teaspoon dried chili flakes
- ½ teaspoon ground black pepper
- 1 carrot, chopped
- 1 garlic clove, pressed
- 2 teaspoon coconut oil
- 3 cups celery, chopped
- 3 cups roasted vegetable broth
- Kosher salt, to taste

Directions:
1. Simply throw all of the above ingredients into your Instant Pot; gently stir until blended. Secure the lid.
2. Choose "Soup/Broth" mode and High pressure; cook for about twenty-five minutes.
3. Once cooking is complete, use a quick pressure release; cautiously remove the lid.
4. Ladle into four soup bowls and serve hot. Enjoy!

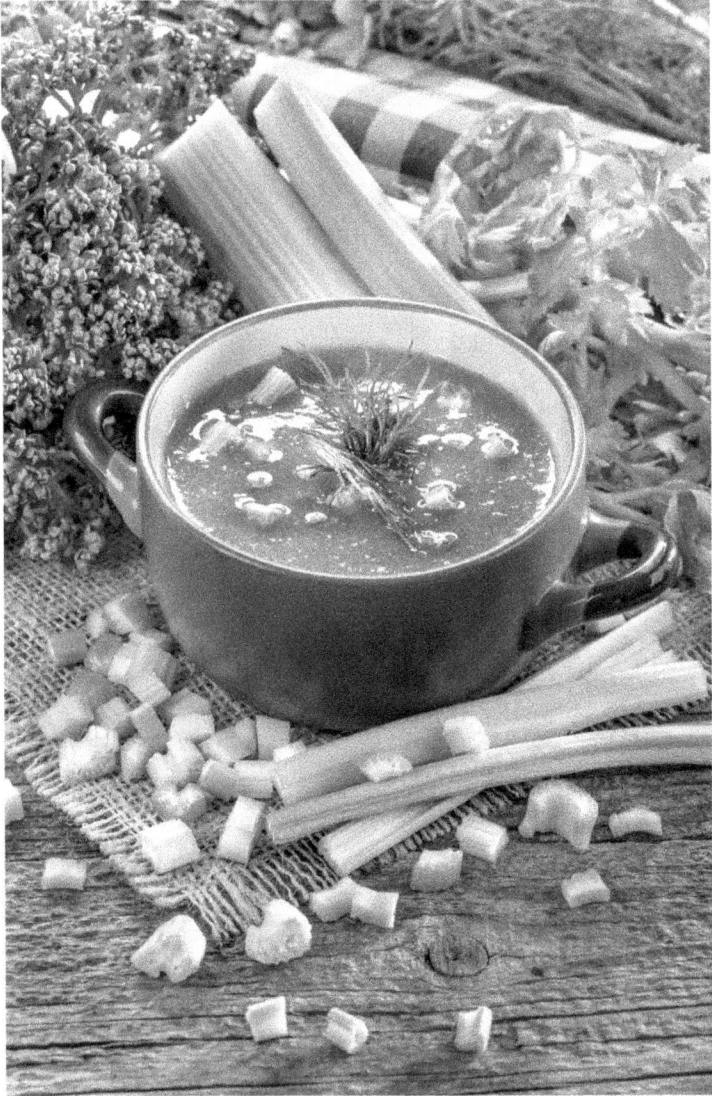

Cheesy Chicken Soup

Time To Prepare: twenty minutes
Time to Cook: 33-40 minutes
Yield: Servings 6

Ingredients:
- ¼ teaspoon black pepper
- ½ cup shredded cheddar cheese
- ½ teaspoon cumin
- ½ teaspoon salt
- 1 cup whipped cream cheese
- 1 tablespoon coconut oil, for cooking
- 1 teaspoon chili powder
- 1 yellow onion, chopped
- 2 boneless, skinless chicken breasts
- 2 cloves garlic, chopped
- 2 cups chicken broth
- 2 cups water

Directions:
1. Heat a big frying pan on moderate heat with a ½ tablespoon of the coconut oil.
2. Brown the chicken breasts until thoroughly cooked. Set aside.
3. Put the garlic and onion to a big stockpot with the rest of the 1 tablespoon of the coconut oil and sauté until translucent over low to moderate heat. This should take about three to five minutes.
4. Put in this chicken broth and water. Whisk in the cream cheese and keep whisking over low to moderate heat until blended.

5. Put in the spices and bring to its boiling point. While the water is boiling, chop the chicken into bite-sized pieces and put it into the stockpot. Reduce to a simmer and cook for half an hour.

6. Mix in the cheddar cheese before you serve.

Chicken And Cauliflower Curry Stew

Time To Prepare: fifteen minutes
Time to Cook: 4 hours
Yield: Servings 7

Ingredients:
- ¼ cup fresh cilantro, chopped
- ⅓ cup coconut oil
- 1 green bell pepper, chopped
- 1 pound (454 g) cauliflower, chopped into little pieces
- 1.5pounds (680 g) skinless, boneless chicken thighs, cut into bite-sized pieces
- 14 ounces (397 g) unsweetened coconut milk
- 2 tablespoons curry powder
- 2 tablespoons ginger garlic paste
- Salt and ground black pepper, to taste

Directions:
1. Warm half of the coconut oil in a nonstick frying pan on moderate heat, then sauté the garlic ginger paste and curry powder for a few minutes or until aromatic.
2. Put in the chicken pieces, and drizzle with salt and pepper. sauté for another ten minutes or until the chicken is mildly browned.
3. Remove from the frying pan and set aside.
4. Warm another half of coconut oil in the frying pan, then sauté the cauliflower and bell pepper on moderate to high heat for one to two minutes.
5. Then fold in the coconut milk and reduce the heat to low.
6. Cover with lid and stew for about forty-five minutes.

7. Drizzle with salt and pepper, then put in the sautéed chicken.
8. Move the stew to a big platter and serve with cilantro on top as decoration.

Chicken Chili Blanco

Time To Prepare: ten minutes
Time to Cook: twenty minutes
Yield: Servings 4

Ingredients:
- ¼ teaspoon cayenne pepper
- 1 tablespoon ghee
- 1 teaspoon chili powder
- 2 (4- ounce) cans diced mild green chiles with their liquid
  2 scallions, cut
- 2 small onions, chopped
- 2 teaspoons dried oregano
- 4 cups chicken broth or vegetable broth
- 4 cups shredded cooked chicken
- 4 cups white beans, drained and washed well
- 4 teaspoons ground cumin
- 6 garlic cloves, minced

Directions:
1. In a huge soup pot on moderate heat, melt the ghee.
2. Put in the onions and garlic, and sauté for five minutes.
3. Place the chiles, and cook for a couple of minutes, stirring.
4. Mix in the beans, broth, cumin, oregano, chili powder, and cayenne pepper.
5. Heat it until it simmers.
6. Put in the chicken, bring to a simmer, decrease the heat to moderate-low, and cook for about ten minutes.
7. Serve instantly, sprinkled with the scallions.

Chickpea Curry Soup

Time To Prepare: ten minutes
Time to Cook: twenty-five minutes
Yield: Servings 4

Ingredients:
- ¼ cup extra-virgin olive oil or coconut oil
- 1 (fifteen-ounce) can chickpeas, drained and washed
- 1 big apple, cored, peeled, and slice into ¼-inch dice
- 1 cup full-fat coconut milk
- 1 medium onion, finely chopped
- 1 teaspoon salt
- 2 garlic cloves, cut
- 2 tablespoons finely chopped fresh cilantro
- 2 teaspoons curry powder
- 3 cups peeled butternut squash cut into ½-inch dice
- 3 cups vegetable broth

Directions:
1. In a large pot, heat the oil on high heat.
2. Put in the onion and garlic and sauté until the onion starts to brown, six to eight minutes. 3. Place the apple, curry powder, and salt and sauté to toast the curry powder, one to two minutes.
4. Place the squash and broth then bring to its boiling point.
5. Reduce the heat then cook until the squash is soft for about ten minutes.
6. Mix in the coconut milk.
7.Use an immersion blender to purée the soup in the pot until the desired smoothness is achieved.

8.Mix in the chickpeas and cilantro, heat through for one to two minutes, before you serve.

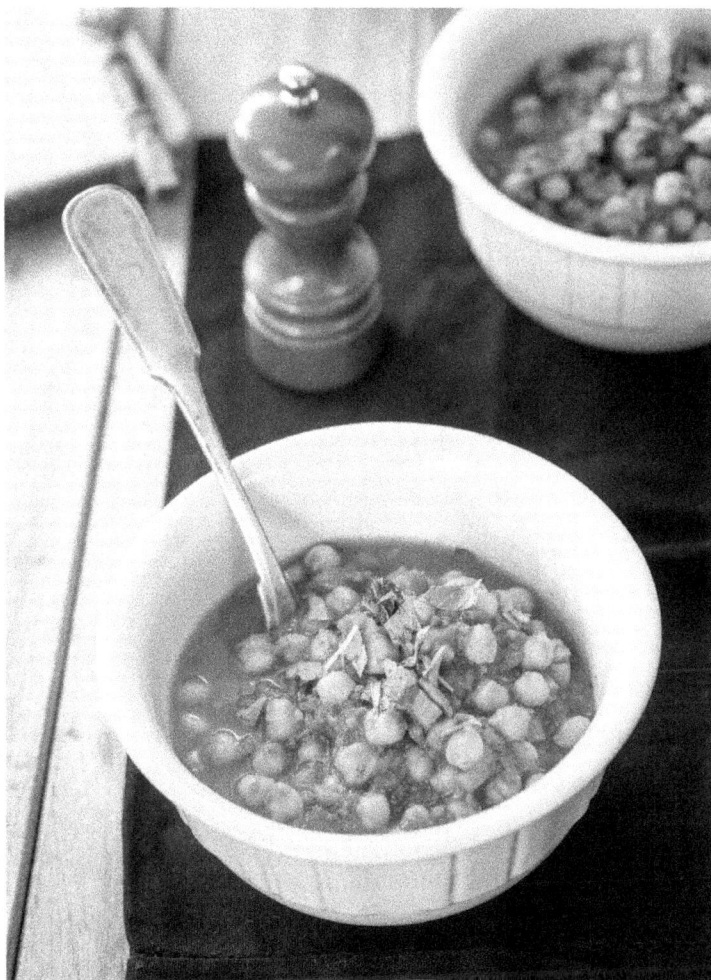

Coconut Cashew Soup with Butternut Squash

Time ToPrepare: ten minutes
Time to Cook: twenty minutes
Yield: Servings 6

Ingredients:

- ½ tsp. salt
- ¾ cup toasted cashews
- 1 (14-ounce) can full-fat coconut milk
- 1 cup mung bean sprouts
- 1 small butternut squash, halved, diced
- 1 small Napa cabbage, shredded
- 1 white onion, diced
- 1½ tbsp. Ginger, peeled and minced
- 2 carrots, chopped
- 2 cups green beans, trimmed
- 2 red chili peppers, seeded and diced
- 2 tbsp. coconut oil
- 3 cups vegetable broth
- 3 garlic cloves, peeled and minced
- 4 tablespoons toasted coconut shavings
- Freshly ground black pepper

Directions:

1. In a huge soup pot on moderate heat, melt the coconut oil.
2. Place the cashews and sauté for a couple of minutes.
3. Take off from the pan and save for later.

4.Place the peppers, garlic, and onion, and sauté for minimum 6 minutes.

5. Then put the ginger and carrots, and sauté for minimum 3 minutes, or until the carrots and squash start to become tender.

6. Stir in the cabbage, green beans, broth, coconut milk, and salt, flavor with pepper.

7.Simmer for fifteen minutes.

8. Remove the heat.

9. Mix in the bean sprouts and coconut shavings.

10. Pour into soup bowls and serve instantly.

Cream of Mushroom Soup

Time To Prepare: twenty minutes
Time to Cook: thirty minutes
Yield: Servings 6

Ingredients:

- 5 cups mushrooms (cut)
- 1 tablespoon sherry
- 3 tablespoons butter
- 3 tablespoons flour
- 1 cup half-and-half Salt
- Ground black pepper
- 1½ cups chicken broth
- ½ cup onion (chopped)
- 1/8 teaspoon dried thyme

Directions:

1. Cook mushrooms with onion and thyme in the broth until soft.
2. Puree the mixture.
3. Whisk some flour in a pan of melted butter.
4. Put in half-and-half, vegetable puree, and seasoning.
5. Boil until it becomes thick.
6. Put in sherry.

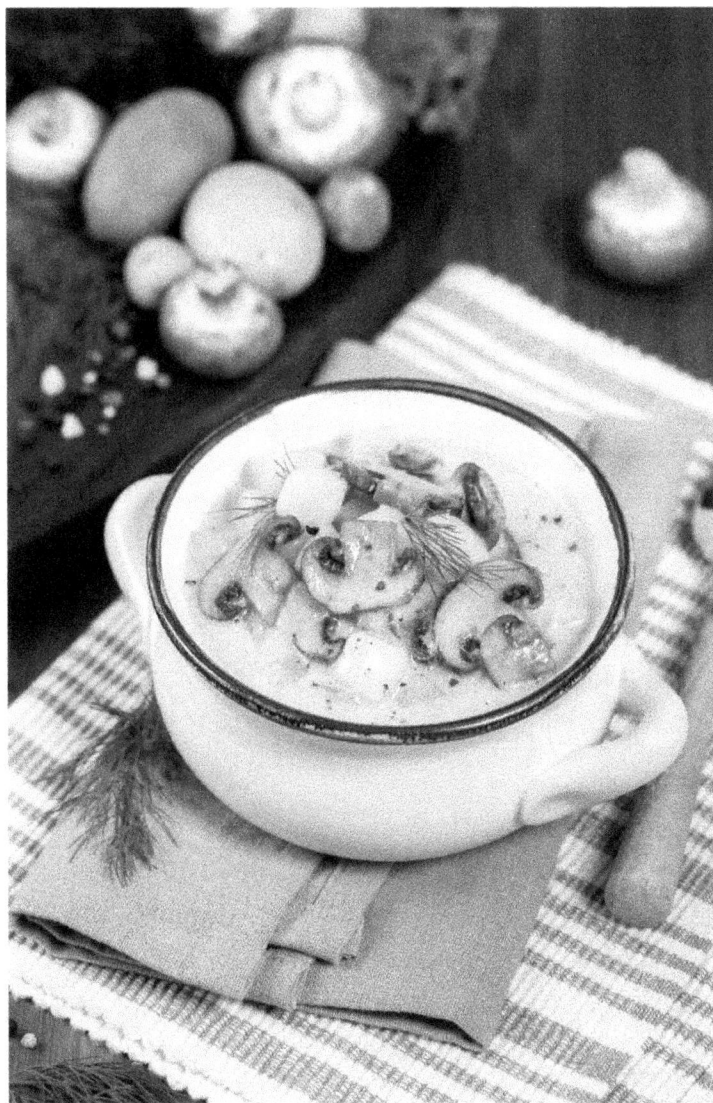

Creamy Broccoli Soup

Time To Prepare: fifteen minutes
Time to Cook: 4 hours
Yield: Servings 7

Ingredients:

- ¼ teaspoon ground black pepper
- ½ teaspoon paprika powder
- ½ teaspoon salt
- ⅔ cup heavy whipping cream
- 1 pinch cayenne pepper
- 1 red onion, roughly chopped
- 1 tablespoon olive oil
- 2 cups chicken broth
- 20 ounces (567 g) broccoli, cut into stalks and florets
- 3 garlic cloves, chopped
- 3 tablespoons butter ounces
- (99 g) Cheddar cheese, shredded

Directions:

1. Warm 1 tablespoon of butter and olive oil in a deep cooking pan, then fry the broccoli stalks and chopped onion on moderate heat for five minutes until soft.
2. Put in the garlic and keep frying for a couple of minutes until mildly browned, then drizzle with cayenne pepper, paprika, salt, and ground black pepper.
3. Cook for another one minutes.
4. Pour over the chicken broth.
5. Cover the lid and leave to simmer for five minutes.

6. Take away the cooked vegetables from the deep cooking pan to a food processor and process.

7. Lightly ladle the soup into the food processor while processing until creamy.

8. Melt the rest of the butter in the deep cooking pan, and fry the broccoli florets for five minutes until tender and soft.

9. Pour the soup from the food processor into the deep cooking pan.

10. Blend to mix thoroughly. If the soup is too thick, you can put in some water to make it thinner.

11. Bring the soup to its boiling point, then reduce the heat and bring to a simmer using low heat for about three minutes.

12. Put in the Cheddar cheese and heavy whipping cream and cook for a couple of minutes more until the cheese melts.

13. Take away the soup from the deep cooking pan and serve warm.

Creamy Leek Soup

Time To Prepare: two minutes
Time to Cook: 8 minutes
Yield: Servings 4

Ingredients:
- ½ cup heavy cream
- ½ cup Monterey-Jack cheese, shredded
- ½ cup tomato purée
- ½ pound chorizo, cut
- 1 bay leaf
- 1 cup leeks, chopped
- 1 green chili, deseeded and finely chopped
- 1 tablespoon sesame oil
- 2 chicken bouillon cubes
- 2 cloves garlic, minced
- 4 cups water

Directions:
1. Push the "Sauté" button to heat up your Instant Pot.
2. Once hot, heat the oil and sauté the leeks until soft.
3. Now, mix in chorizo, garlic, and green chili; carry on cooking until aromatic.
4. Next, put in water, tomato puree, heavy cream, bouillon cubes, and bay leaf.
5. Secure the lid.
6. Choose "Manual" mode and High pressure; cook for about six minutes.
7. Once cooking is complete, use a natural pressure release; cautiously remove the lid.

8. Next, press the "Sauté" button and put in the cheese; allow it to simmer until the cheese is melted and thoroughly heated

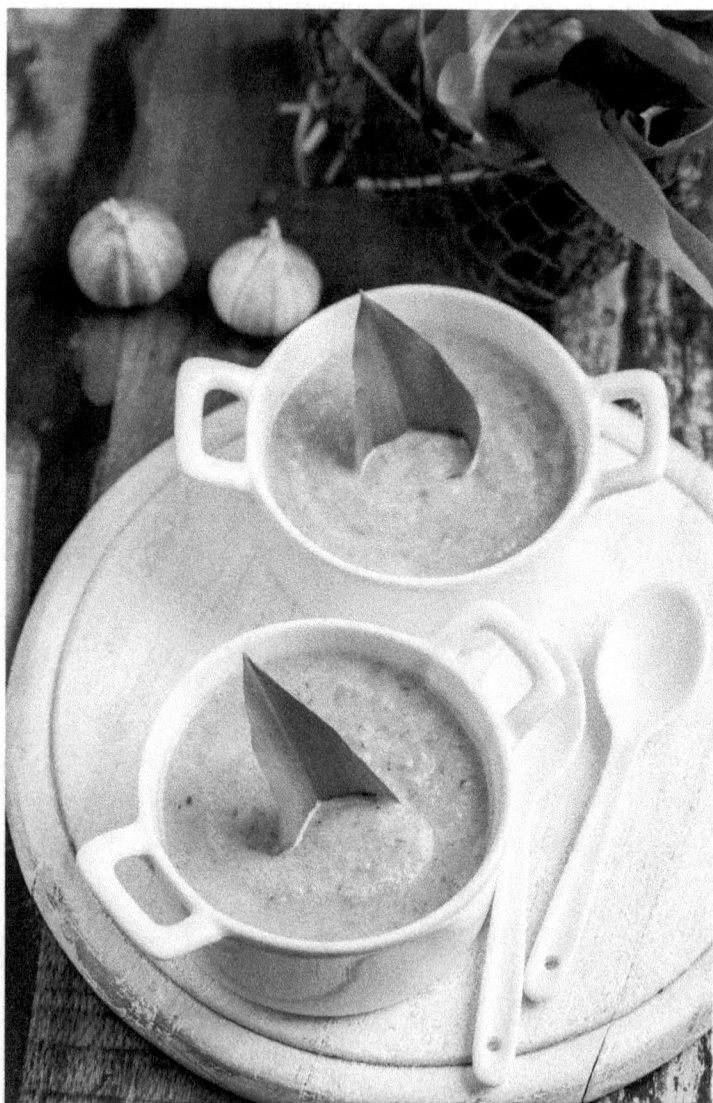

Creamy Pumpkin Puree Soup

Time To Prepare: ten minutes
Time to Cook: forty-five minutes
Yield: Servings 3

Ingredients:
- 1 cup Heavy Cream
- 1 cup Pumpkin puree
- 2 cups Chicken broth
- 2 tbsp. Olive oil
- 4-5 Garlic cloves
- Salt and black pepper to taste

Directions:
1. In the Instant Pot, put in all ingredients.
2. Secure the lid and cook for forty minutes on Meat/Stew mode on High.
3. When ready, press Cancel and do a quick pressure release.
4. Move to a blender and blend thoroughly.
5. Pour into serving bowls to serve

Creamy Turmeric Cauliflower Soup

Time To Prepare: ten minutes
Time to Cook: fifteen minutes
Yield: Servings 4

Ingredients:

- ¼ cup finely chopped fresh cilantro
- ¼ teaspoon freshly ground black pepper
- ¼ teaspoon ground cumin
- ½ teaspoon salt
- 1 (1¼-inch) piece fresh ginger, peeled and cut
- 1 cup full-fat coconut milk
- 1 garlic clove, peeled
- 1 leek, white part only, thinly cut
- 1½ teaspoons turmeric
- 2 tablespoons extra-virgin olive oil
- 3 cups cauliflower florets
- 3 cups vegetable broth

Directions:

1. In a large pot, heat the oil on high heat.
2. Put in the leek, and sauté until it just starts to brown, three to four minutes.
3. Put in the cauliflower, garlic, ginger, turmeric, salt, pepper, and cumin and sauté to lightly toast the spices, one to two minutes.
4. Pour the broth then bring to its boiling point.
5. Reduce the heat and cook until the cauliflower is soft for about five minutes.

6. Use an immersion blender to purée the soup in the pot until the desired smoothness is achieved.

7.Stir in the coconut milk and cilantro, heat through, before you serve.

Detox Cabbage Soup

Time To Prepare: ten minutes
Time to Cook: thirty-five minutes
Yield: Servings 4

Ingredients:
- 1 tbs. freshly grated ginger root
- 2 big carrot
- 1 cup whole canned tomatoes with juice
- 1 whole head of cabbage
- 1 tbs. freshly grated turmeric root
- 3 celery stalks with leaves
- Enough water to immerse the vegetables
- 2 medium Russet potatoes
- Sea salt & black pepper to taste
- ½ medium onion
- 1/4 cup extra virgin olive oil

Directions:

1. Heat the oil in a large pot on moderate heat for a couple of minutes.

2. Put in the celery, onions, ginger, carrots & turmeric, then sauté on medium until translucent.

3. Sprinkle with salt & pepper to taste.

4. With the heat still on moderate, dice the potatoes & generally slash the cabbage at that point put into the pot alongside the whole tomatoes & juice.

5. While they cook, separate the tomatoes using a fork or blade.

6. Fill the pot with sufficient water to simply cover the cabbage.

7. Cover with a top & heat to the point of boiling.

8. When bubbling, evacuate the top & cook for around thirty minutes or until the potatoes & cabbage are fork delicate.
9. Put in the ice chest for as long as 5 days & in the cooler for as long as three months.

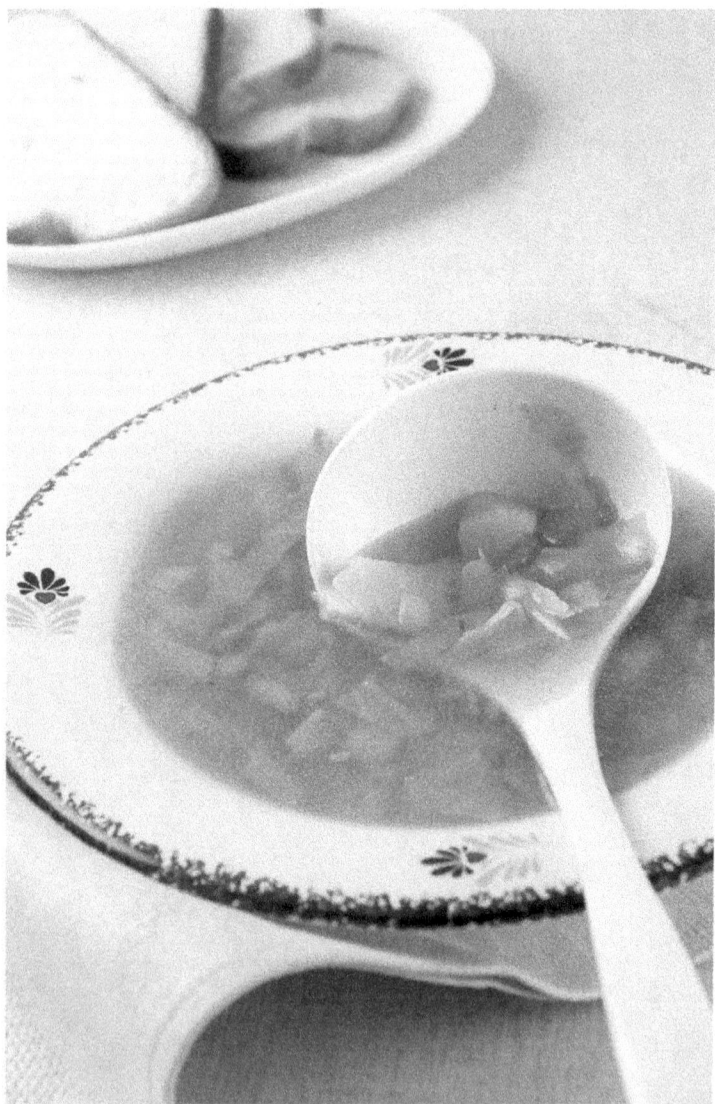

French Caramelized Onion Soup

Time To Prepare: five minutes
Time to Cook: ten minutes
Yield: Servings 4

Ingredients:

- ½ stick butter, softened
- 4 cups chicken stock
- ½ teaspoon dried basil
- Kosher salt and ground black pepper, to taste
- ½ cup Swiss cheese, freshly grated
- 3/4 pound yellow onions, cut

Directions:

1. Push the "Sauté" button to heat up your Instant Pot. Once hot, melt the butter and sauté the onions until caramelized and soft.

2. Put in chicken stock, basil, salt, and black pepper. Secure the lid. Choose "Manual" mode and High pressure; cook for about ten minutes.

3. Once cooking is complete, use a quick pressure release; cautiously remove the lid.

4. Ladle the soup into separate bowls and top with grated cheese.

5. Enjoy

Garlic Mushroom & Beef Soup

Time To Prepare: ten minutes
Time to Cook: forty minutes
Yield: Servings 6

Ingredients:
- ½ cup heavy cream cup whipped cream cheese
- 1 pound beef chuck, cubed
- 1 tablespoon coconut oil, for cooking
- 1 yellow onion, chopped
- 1½ cups cremini mushrooms
- 2 cloves garlic, chopped
- 6 cups beef broth
- Salt & pepper, to taste

Directions:
1. Put in the coconut oil to a frying pan and brown the beef.
2. Once cooked, put in the beef to the base of a stockpot with all of the ingredients minus the heavy cream.
3. Mix thoroughly.
4. Heat to a simmer and whisk again until the cream cheese is mixed uniformly into the soup.
5. Cook for half an hour Warm the heavy cream, and then put in to the soup

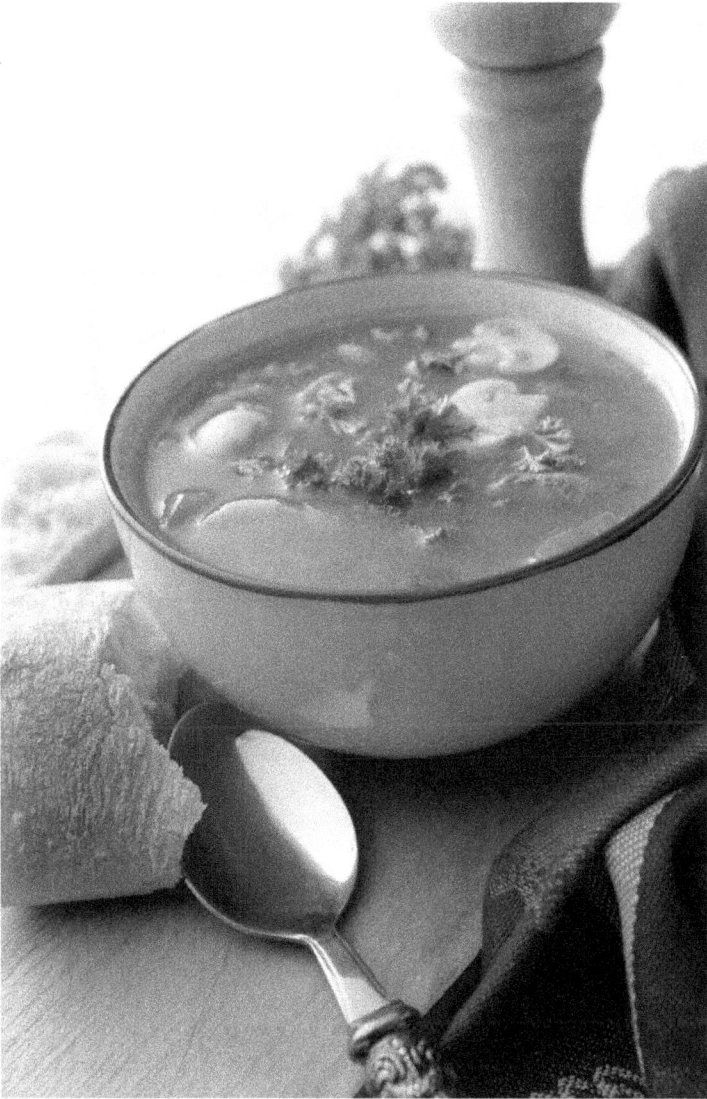

Golden Chickpea And Vegetable Soup

Time To Prepare: fifteen minutes
Time to Cook: twenty minutes
Yield: Servings 6

Ingredients:

- 1 ½ cup Diced celery
- 1 ½ cup Sliced leeks
- 1 cup cooked chickpeas
- 1 cup diced carrots
- 1 cup Torn curly kale leaves
- 1 tbsp. Grated ginger
- 2 cloves minced garlic
- 2 cups Cauliflower florets
- 2 tbsp. Curry powder
- 2 tbsp. Minced organic parsley
- 2 tsp. Coconut oil
- 4 cups Bone broth

Directions:
1. Warm the coconut oil in a pot and put in the garlic and ginger.
2. Sauté for one minute before you put in the turmeric and curry powder and sautéing for one more minute.
3. Throw in celery, leeks, carrots, and cauliflower, continuously stirring for approximately one minute.
4. Put in the bone broth and chickpeas.
5. Cover the pot and leave to boil.

6. Reduce the heat and allow it to simmer for minimum fifteen minutes.

7. Turn off heat and put in parsley and kale, leaving the heat to cook the leaves.

8. Drizzle salt and pepper. Serve

Mixed Veggies Stew

Yield: 4 servings
Preparation Time: fifteen minutes
Cooking Time: 21 minutes

Ingredients:
- 2 tablespoons coconut oil
- 1 large onion, chopped
- 1 teaspoon ground turmeric
- 1 teaspoon ground cumin
- Salt and freshly ground black pepper, to taste
- 1-2 cups water, divided
- 1 cup cabbage, shredded
- 1 bunch broccoli, chopped
- 2 large carrots, peeled and sliced
- 2 teaspoons fresh ginger, grated

Directions:
1. In a large soup pan, melt coconut oil on medium heat.
2. Add onion and sauté approximately 5 minutes.
3. Stir in spices and sauté for about 1 minute.
4. Add 1 cup of water and convey to some boil.
5. Simmer for approximately 10 min.
6. Add vegetables and enough water that covers the 50 % of vegetables mixture.
7. Simmer, covered for about 10-fifteen minutes, stirring occasionally.
8. Serve hot.

Chicken & Tomato Stew

Yield: 6-8 servings
Preparation Time: fifteen minutes
Cooking Time: 31 minutes

Ingredients:
- 2 tablespoons olive oil
- 1 onion, chopped
- ½ tablespoon fresh ginger, grated finely
- 1 tablespoon fresh garlic, minced
- 1 teaspoon ground turmeric
- 1 teaspoon ground cumin
- 1 teaspoon ground coriander
- 1 teaspoon paprika
- 1 teaspoon red pepper cayenne
- 6 skinless, boneless chicken thighs, trimmed and cut into 1-inch pieces
- 3 Roma tomatoes, chopped
- 1 (14-ounce) coconut milk
- Salt and freshly ground black pepper, to taste
- 1/3 cup fresh cilantro, chopped

Directions:
1. In a substantial pan, heat oil on medium heat.
2. Add onion and sauté for around 8-10 minutes.
3. Add ginger, garlic and spices and sauté for approximately 1 minute.
4. Add chicken and cook for around 4-5 minutes.
5. Add tomatoes, coconut milk, salt and black pepper and bring to a gentle simmer.

6. Reduce the heat to low and simmer, covered for around 10-15 minutes or till desired doneness.

7. Stir in cilantro and take away from heat.

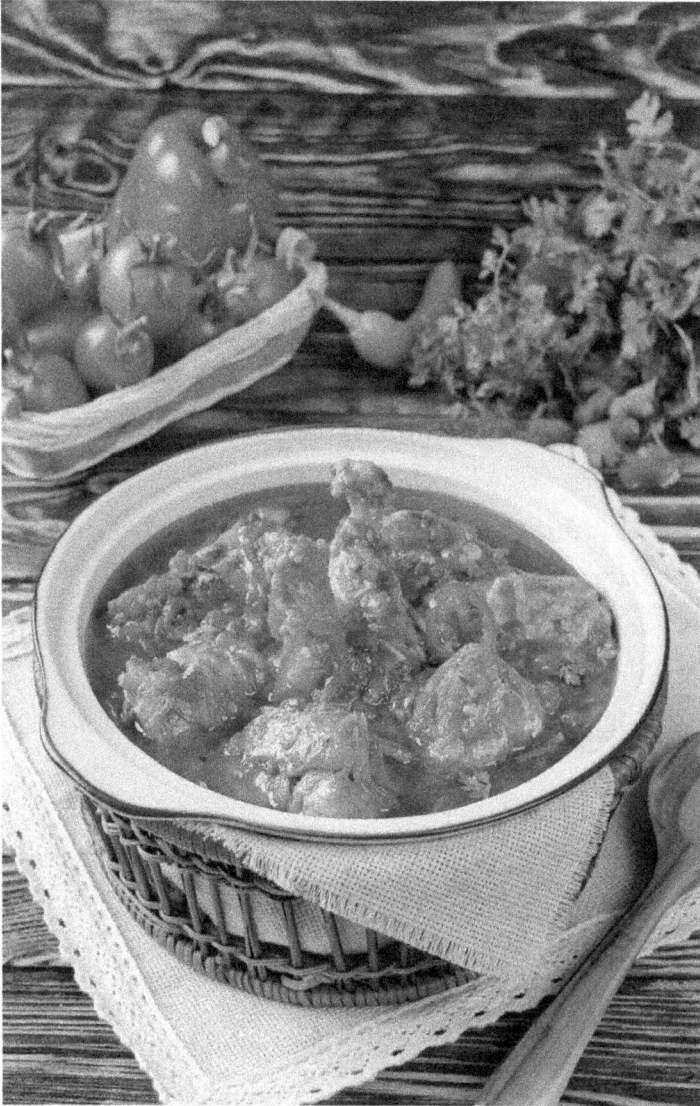

Beef & Squash Stew

Yield: 4-6 servings
Preparation Time: fifteen minutes
Cooking Time: 60 minutes 17 minutes

Ingredients:

- 1½ tablespoons coconut oil, divided
- 2-3 pound stew meat, trimmed and cubed into 1½-inch size
- 1 onion, chopped
- 1 (2-inch) piece fresh ginger, minced
- 5 garlic cloves, minced
- 2 cups bone broth
- 1 butternut squash, peeled and cubed
- ¼ teaspoon ground cinnamon
- 2 pears, cored and chopped
- 1 cup fresh mushrooms, sliced
- 1 tablespoon fresh thyme, chopped

Directions:

1. In a big heavy bottomed pan, heat 1 tablespoon of oil on medium-high heat
2. Add beef and sear for around 8-10 minutes or till browned completely.
3. With a slotted spoon, transfer the beef into a bowl.
4. Now, decrease the heat to medium.
5. Add onion and sauté for approximately 5 minutes.
6. Add ginger and garlic and sauté for about 2 minutes.
7. Add cooked beef and broth and provide with a boil.

8. Reduce the warmth to low and simmer, covered approximately 15 minutes.

9. Stir in squash, cinnamon and salt and simmer, covered for around fifteen minutes.

10. Stir in pears and simmer, covered for approximately half an hour.

11. Meanwhile in the small skillet, heat the remaining oil on high heat.

12. Add mushrooms and cook for approximately 5 minutes or till browned.

13. Serve the stew with the topping of mushrooms and thyme.

Haddock & Potato Stew

Yield: 4 servings
Preparation Time: 15 minutes
Cooking Time: 13 minutes

Ingredients:
- 2 large Yukon Gold potatoes, sliced into ¼-inch size
- 1 tbsp olive oil
- 1 (2- inch) piece fresh ginger, chopped finely
- 1 (16-ounce) can whole tomatoes, crushed
- ½ cup water
- 1 cup clam juice
- ¼ teaspoon red pepper flakes, crushed
- Salt, to taste
- 1½ pound boneless haddock, cut into 2inch pieces
- 2 tablespoons fresh parsley, chopped

Direction:
1. Arrange a steamer basket in a big pan of water and produce to your boil.
2. Place the potatoes in the steamer basket and cook, covered approximately 8 minutes.
3. Meanwhile in the pan, heat oil on medium heat.
4. Add ginger and sauté for about 1 minute.
5. Add tomatoes and cook, stirring continuously approximately 2 minutes.
6. Add water, clam juice, red pepper flakes and produce to a boil.
7. Simmer for around 5 minutes, stirring occasionally.

8. Gently, stir in haddock pieces and simmer, covered for about 5 minutes or till desired doneness.

9. In serving bowls, divide potatoes and top with haddock mixture.

10. Garnish with parsley and serve.

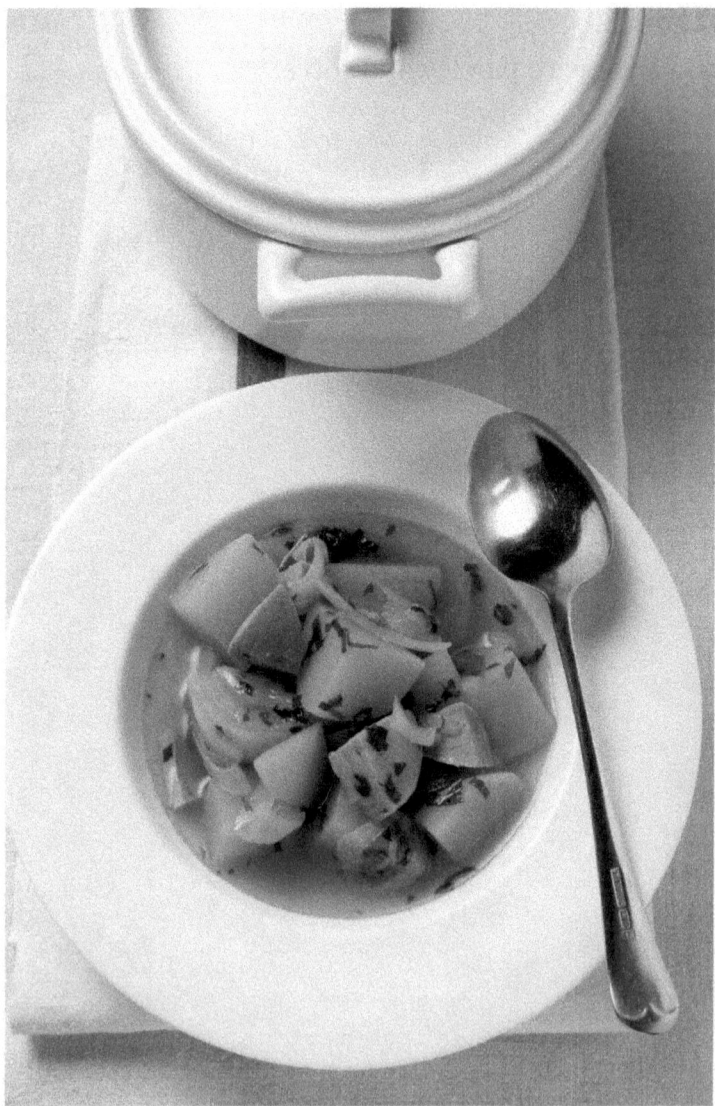

Black-Eyed Beans Stew

Yield: 4-5 servings
Preparation Time: 15 minutes
Cooking Time: 120 minutes 20 min

Ingredients:

- 2 cups dried black eyed beans, soaked for overnight, rinsed and drained
- 2 medium onions, chopped and divided
- 1 (4-inch) piece fresh ginger chopped
- 4 garlic cloves, chopped
- ¼ cup essential olive oil
- 2 scotch bonnet peppers
- 2 (14-ounce) cans plum tomatoes
- ½-¾ cup water
- 1 vegetable bouillon cube
- Salt, to taste

Directions:

1. In a big pan of boiling water, add beans and cook, covered approximately 60-90 minutes or till beans become soft.
2. In a blender, add 1 onion, ginger and garlic and pulse till a puree forms.
3. In a big pan, heat oil on medium heat.
4. Add onion and sauté for around 2-5 minutes.
5. Stir in 5 tablespoons of onion puree and cook for approximately 5 minutes.
6. Meanwhile in a blender, add bonnet peppers and tomatoes and pulse till smooth.
7. Add tomato mixture and stir to blend.

8. Reduce the warmth to low and simmer, covered for about 30 minutes, stirring occasionally.

9. Stir in beans, cube and salt and simmer for approximately 10 minutes.

Lentil Stew

Yield: 4 servings
Preparation Time: quarter-hour
Cooking Time: 50 minutes

Ingredients:
- 1 cup dry lentils, rinsed and drained
- 1 cup potato, peeled and chopped
- ½ cup celery, chopped
- ½ cup carrot, peeled and chopped
- ½ cup onion, chopped
- 1 garlic cloves, minced
- 1 (14½-ounce) peeled Italian tomatoes, chopped
- 1 tablespoon dried basil, crushed
- 1 tablespoon dried parsley, crushed
- Freshly ground black pepper, to taste
- 3½ cups chicken broth

Directions:
1. In a big pan, add all ingredients and stir to blend.
2. Bring with a boil on high heat.
3. Reduce heat to low and simmer, covered approximately 45-50 minutes, stirring occasionally.

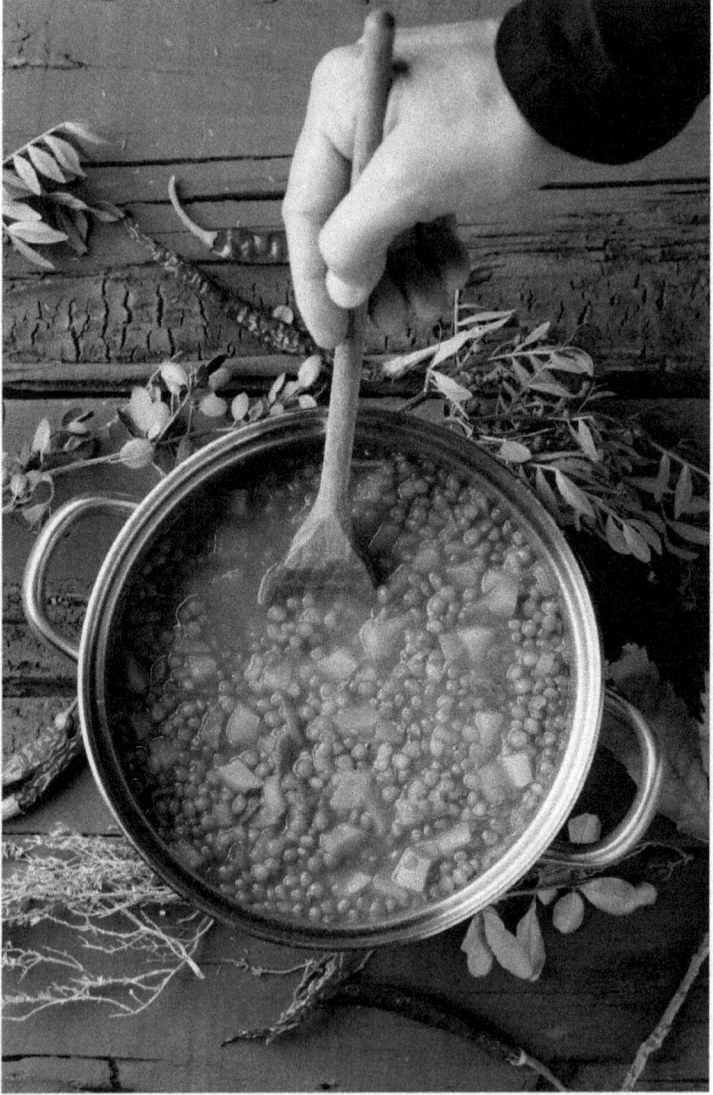

Green Blast Soup

Time To Prepare: ten minutes
Time to Cook: twenty minutes
Yield: Servings 4

Ingredients:

- ¼ cup chopped cashews (not necessary)
- ¼ cup extra-virgin olive oil
- ¼ teaspoon freshly ground black pepper
- 1 bunch Swiss chard, crudely chopped
- 1 fennel bulb, trimmed and thinly cut
- 1 garlic clove, peeled
- 1 teaspoon salt 2 leeks, white parts only, thinly cut
- 2 tablespoons apple cider vinegar
- 3 cups vegetable broth
- 4 cups crudely chopped kale
- 4 cups crudely chopped mustard greens

Directions:

1. In a large pot, heat the oil on high heat.

2. Put in the leeks, fennel, and garlic and sauté until tender, for approximately five minutes.

3. Put in the Swiss chard, kale, and mustard greens and sauté until the greens wilt, two to three minutes.

4. Pour the broth then bring to its boiling point.

5. Reduce the heat to a simmer and cook until the vegetables are completely tender and soft about five minutes.

6. Mix in the vinegar, salt, pepper, and cashews (if using).

7. Use an immersion blender to purée the soup in the pot until the desired smoothness is achieved before you serve.

Hamburger & Tomato Soup

Time To Prepare: ten minutes
Time to Cook: 4 hours
Yield: Servings 6

Ingredients:

- ½ cup beef broth
- ½ cup no-sugar added marinara sauce
- ½ cup shredded cheddar cheese
- 1 pound lean ground beef
- 1 yellow onion, chopped
- 2 cloves garlic, chopped
- Salt & pepper, to taste

Directions:

1. Put all the ingredients in a slow cooker minus the shredded cheese and cook on high for 4 hours.
2. Mix in the cheese before you serve

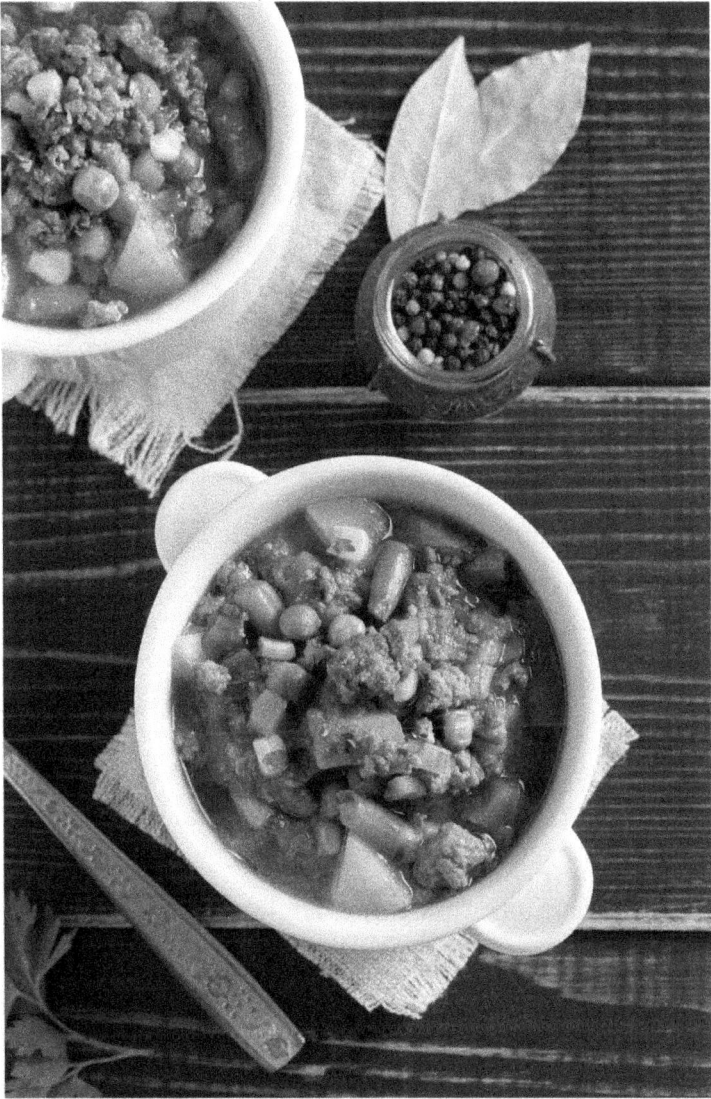

Hearty Root Vegetable Soup

Time To Prepare: five minutes
Time to Cook: ten minutes
Yield: Servings 4

Ingredients:

- 1 bay leaf
- 1 carrot, cut
- 1 celery, diced
- 1 garlic clove, minced
- 1 parsnip, cut
- 1 tablespoon fresh parsley, roughly chopped
- 1 teaspoon fresh sage
- 2 cups cauliflower, cut into little florets
- 4 cups chicken stock
- 4 tablespoons olive oil
- Kosher salt and freshly ground black pepper, to taste

Directions:

1. Simply drop all of the above ingredients into your Instant Pot. Secure the lid.
2. Choose "Manual" mode and High pressure; cook for about ten minutes.
3. Once cooking is complete, use a natural pressure release; cautiously remove the lid.
4. Taste, calibrate the seasonings and serve instantly. Enjoy!

Italian Beef Soup

Time To Prepare: ten minutes
Time to Cook: 4 hours
Yield: Servings 6

Ingredients:
- ½ cup diced tomatoes
- ½ cup shredded mozzarella cheese
- 1 cup beef broth
- 1 cup heavy cream
- 1 pound lean ground beef
- 1 tablespoon Italian seasoning
- 1 yellow onion, chopped
- 2 cloves garlic, chopped
- Salt & pepper, to taste

Directions:
1. Put all the ingredients in a slow cooker minus the heavy cream and mozzarella cheese.
2. Cook on high for 4 hours.
3. Warm the heavy cream, and then put in the warmed cream and cheese to the soup.
4. Stir thoroughly before you serve.

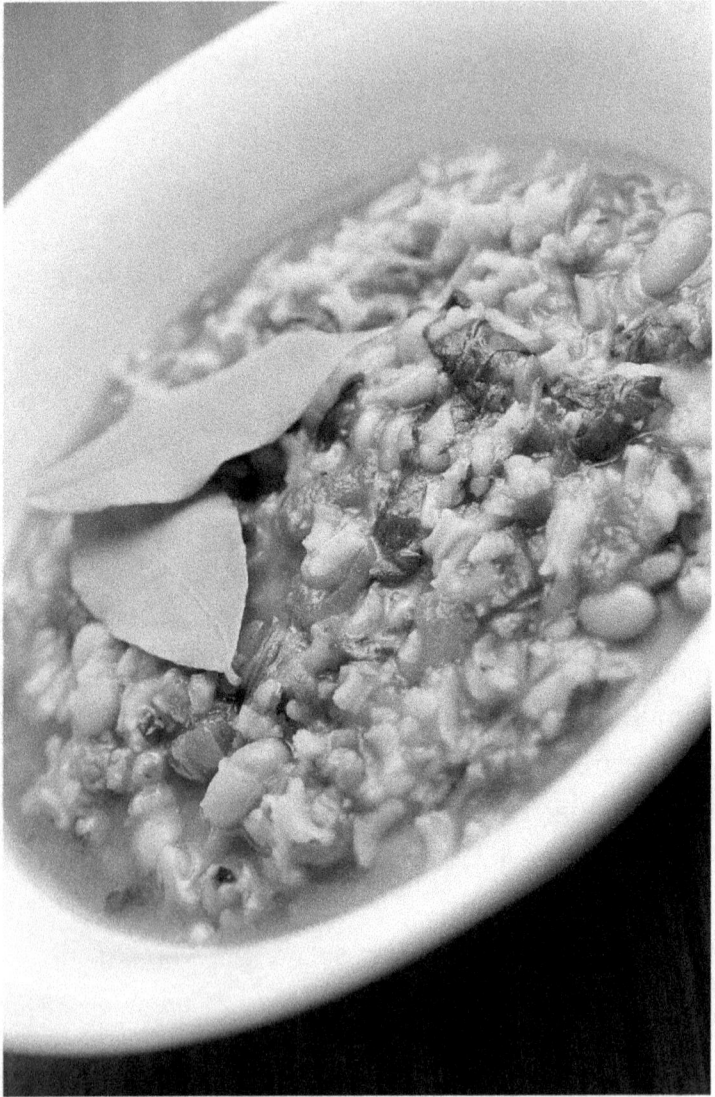

Sugars Italian Summer Squash Soup

Time To Prepare: ten minutes
Time to Cook: fifteen minutes
Yield: Servings 4

Ingredients:
- ½ cup shredded carrot
- 1 cup shredded yellow squash
- 1 cup shredded zucchini
- 1 garlic clove, minced
- 1 small red onion, thinly cut
- 1 tablespoon finely chopped fresh chives
- 1 teaspoon salt
- 2 tablespoons finely chopped fresh basil
- 2 tablespoons pine nuts
- 3 cups vegetable broth
- 3 tablespoons extra-virgin olive oil

Directions:
1. In a large pot, heat the oil using high heat.
2. Put in the onion and garlic and sauté until tender, five to seven minutes.
3. Put in the zucchini, yellow squash, and carrot and sauté until tender, one to two minutes.
4. Pour the broth and salt then bring to its boiling point.
5. Reduce the heat and cook until the vegetables are soft, one to two minutes.
6. Mix in the basil and chives and serve, sprinkled with the pine nuts

Lamb Stew

Time To Prepare: five minutes
Time to Cook: 8 hours
Yield: Servings 6

Ingredients:
- 1 lamb stock cube
- 1 onion, roughly chopped
- 2 pounds (907 g) boneless lamb, cut into cubes
- 2 tablespoons olive oil, plus more for greasing the frying pan
- 2 teaspoons dried rosemary
- 3 cups water
- 4 garlic cloves, finely chopped

From the cupboard:
- Salt and freshly ground black pepper, to taste

Directions:
1. Position the lamb into a mildly greased nonstick frying pan, and cook using high heat for a couple of minutes or until browned.
2. Grease a slow cooker with olive oil, then put in the cooked lamb, stock cube, rosemary, onion, garlic, salt, black pepper, and 3 cups of water.
3. Blend to blend well.
4. Place the slow cooker lid on and cook on LOW for eight hours.
5. Take away the cooked lamb stew from the slow cooker and serve warm.

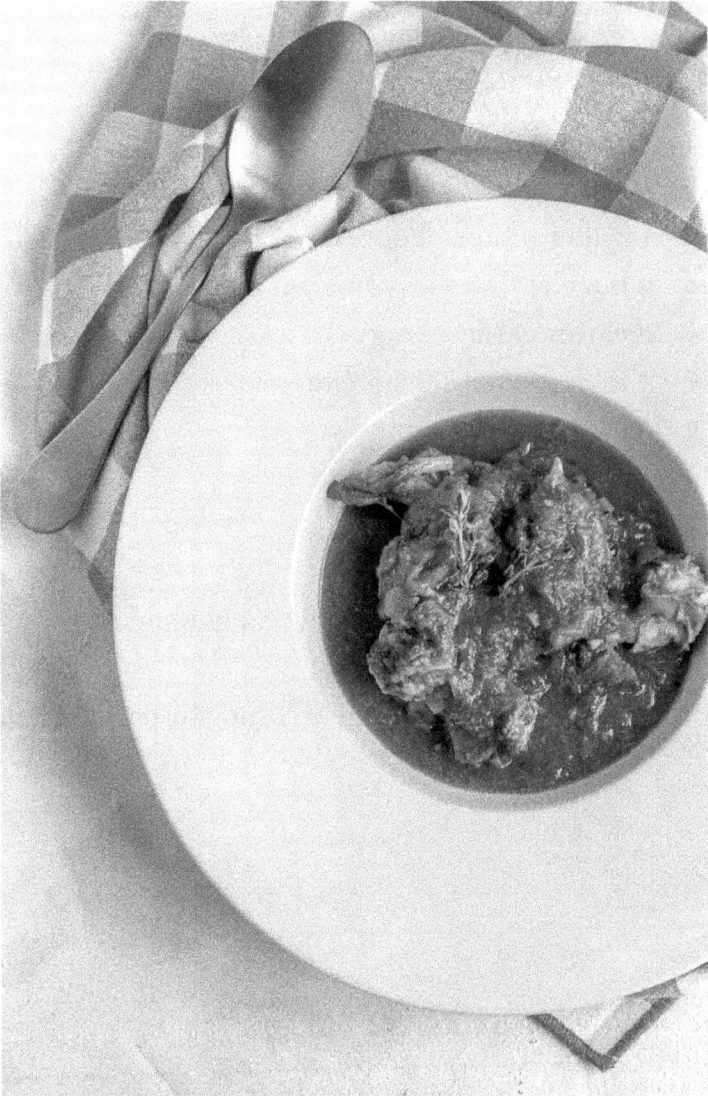

Lemon Chicken Soup

Time To Prepare: ten minutes
Time to Cook: 4 hours
Yield: Servings 4

Ingredients:

- ¼ cup freshly squeezed lemon juice
- 1 yellow onion, chopped
- 2 boneless, skinless chicken breasts
- 2 cloves garlic, chopped
- 2 tablespoons chives, chopped
- 6 cups chicken broth
- Salt & pepper, to taste

Directions:

1. Put all the ingredients in a slow cooker and cook on high for 4 hours.

2. Once cooked, shred the chicken and stir back into the soup

Minestrone Soup with Quinoa

Time To Prepare: ten minutes
Time to Cook: twenty minutes
Yield: Servings 6

Ingredients:
- ½ cup quinoa, washed well
- ½ red bell pepper, diced
- ½ teaspoon salt
- 1 (14 oz.) can cannellini beans, drained and washed well
- 1 (14 oz.) can diced tomatoes with its juice
- 1 bay leaf
- 1 cup packed kale, stemmed and meticulously washed
- 1 medium white onion, diced
- 1 small zucchini, diced
- 1 tablespoon freshly squeezed lemon juice
- 1 tablespoon ghee 2 carrots, chopped
- 2 celery stalks, diced
- 2 garlic cloves, minced
- 2 teaspoons dried rosemary
- 2 teaspoons dried thyme
- 5 cups vegetable broth
- Freshly ground black pepper

Directions:

1. In a huge soup pot on moderate heat, put in the ghee, garlic, onion, carrots, and celery, and sauté for about three minutes.
2. Put in the zucchini and red bell pepper, and sauté for a couple of minutes.

3. Mix in the broth, tomatoes, beans, kale, quinoa, lemon juice, rosemary, thyme, bay leaf, and salt, and flavor with black pepper.

4. Put it to a simmer, reduce the heat temperature, cover, and cook for fifteen minutes, or until the quinoa is cooked.

5. Take away the bay leaf and discard it.

6. Serve hot.

Mushroom And Thyme Soup

TimeTo Prepare: five minutes
Time to Cook: twenty minutes
Yield: Servings 4

Ingredients:
- ¼ cup butter
- 12 ounces (340 g) wild mushrooms, chopped
- 2 garlic cloves, minced
- 2 teaspoons thyme leaves
- 4 cups vegetable broth
- 5 ounces (142 g) crème fraiche

From the cupboard:
- Salt and freshly ground black pepper, to taste

Directions:
1. Place the butter in a deep cooking pan and melt on moderate heat.
2. Put in the minced garlic and cook for a few minutes or until aromatic.
3. Put in the chopped mushrooms, and drizzle with salt and black pepper.
4. Stir to blend and cook for about ten minutes or until the mushrooms are soft.
5. Put in the vegetable broth and bring the soup to its boiling point.
6. Stir continuously.
7. Reduce the heat and simmer the soup for about ten minutes or until it becomes slightly thick.

8. Pour the soup in a blender, and pulse until smooth, then fold in the crème fraiche.

9. Move the soup in a big container and top with thyme leaves before you serve.

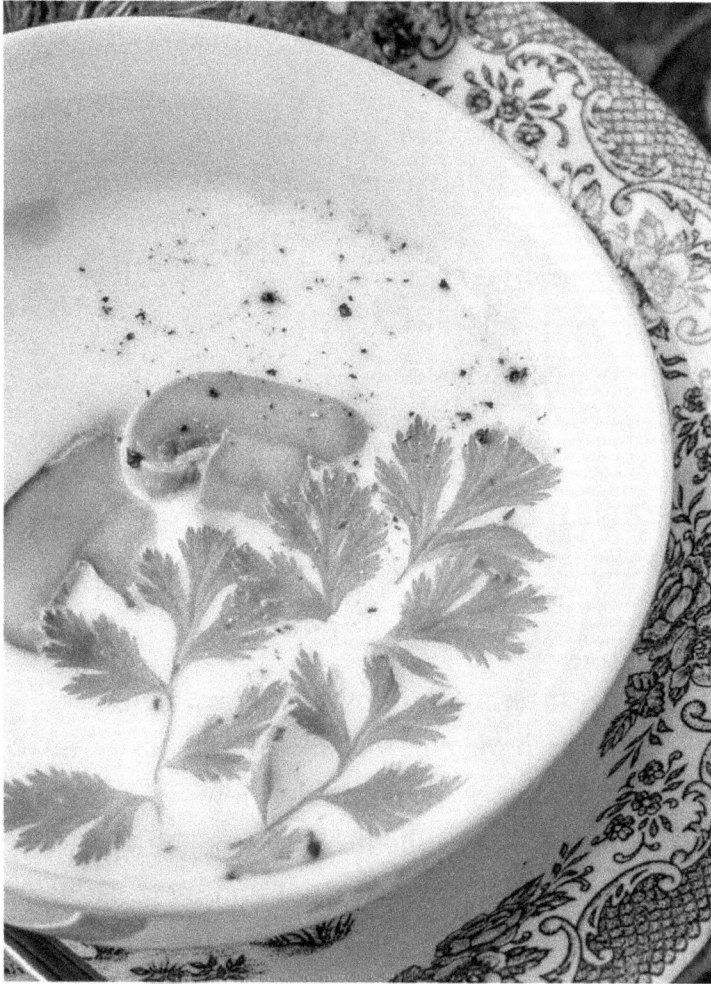

Pork Stew

Time To Prepare: five minutes
Time to Cook: 8 hours
Yield: Servings 6

Ingredients:

- 1 onion, finely chopped
- 1 teaspoon dried mixed spices (homemade or store bought)
- 2 pounds (907 g) pork loin, cut into cubes
- 2 tablespoons olive oil
- 3 cups chicken stock
- 4 garlic cloves, crushed

From the cupboard:

- Salt and freshly ground black pepper, to taste

Directions:

1. Grease the insert of the slow cooker with olive oil.
2. Combine the pork, chicken stock, onion, dried mixed spices, garlic, salt, and black pepper in the slow cooker.
3. Place the slow cooker lid on and cook on LOW for eight hours.
4. Ladle the stew in a big container and serve warm.

Pumpkin, Coconut & Sage Soup

Soup Time To Prepare: fifteen minutes
Time to Cook: thirty minutes
Yield: Servings 6

Ingredients:

- 1 cup canned pumpkin
- 1 cup full-fat coconut milk
- 1 teaspoon freshly chopped sage
- 2 cloves garlic, chopped
- 6 cups vegetable broth
- Pinch of salt & pepper, to taste

Directions:

1. Put in all the ingredients minus the coconut milk to a stockpot on moderate heat and bring to its boiling point.
2.Reduce to a simmer and cook for half an hour.
3. Put in the coconut milk and stir.

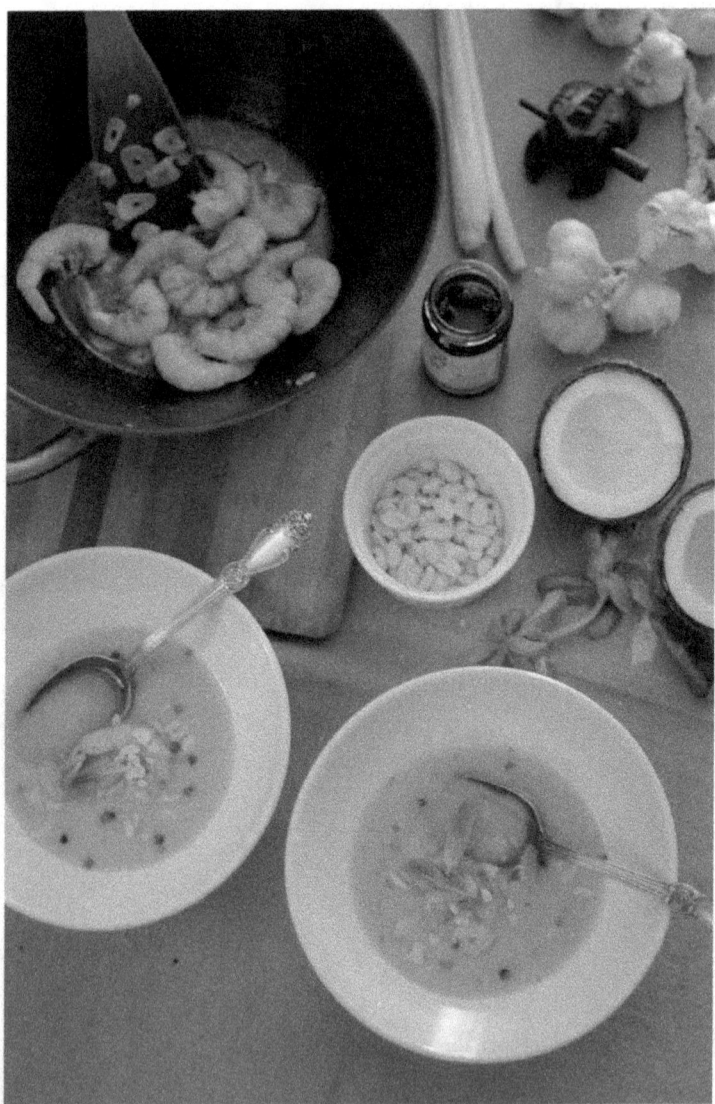

Red Lentil Dal

Time To Prepare: ten minutes
Time to Cook: twenty minutes
Yield: Servings 6

Ingredients:

- ½ teaspoon salt
- 1 (14-ounce) can unsweetened coconut milk
- 1 bay leaf
- 1 cup red dried lentils, sorted and washed well
- 1 medium tomato, diced
- 1 medium white onion, diced
- 1 tablespoon coconut oil
- 1 teaspoon ground cumin
- 1 teaspoon ground ginger
- 1 teaspoon ground turmeric
- 1 teaspoon mustard seeds
- 1 teaspoon sesame seeds
- 2 garlic cloves, minced
- 2 tablespoons chopped fresh cilantro leaves
- 3 cups vegetable broth
- Dash ground cinnamon

Directions:

1. In a huge soup pot using high heat, combine the broth, lentils, and bay leaf, and place to its boiling point.

2. Lessen the heat to moderate-low and simmer for about twenty minutes, or until the lentils are cooked.

3.In the meantime, in a moderate-sized deep cooking pan on moderate heat, sauté the onion and garlic in the coconut oil for a couple of minutes.

4. Put in the tomato, sesame seeds, ginger, cumin, turmeric, mustard seeds, salt, and cinnamon.

5. Cook, regularly stirring, for five minutes.

6. Mix in the coconut milk, then put it to a simmer.

7. Remove and discard the bay leaf.

8. Put in the coconut milk mixture to the lentils together with the cilantro, and stir until blended.

9. Serve alone or over rice if you wish.

Rich Onion And Beef Stew

Time To Prepare: five minutes
Time to Cook: 10 hours
Yield: Servings 6

Ingredients:
- 1 beef stock cube
- 1 teaspoon dried mixed herbs (such as Italian seasoning)
- 2 onions, roughly chopped
- 2 pounds (907 g) boneless stewing beef, cut into cubes
- 3 cups water
- 3 tablespoons olive oil, divided
- 5 garlic cloves, crushed

From the cupboard:
- Salt and freshly ground black pepper, to taste

Directions:
1. Grease the insert of the slow cooker with 2 tablespoons of olive oil.
2. Coat a nonstick frying pan with the rest of the olive oil. Heat the oil in the frying pan on moderate to high heat, then put the beef in the frying pan and sear for a couple of minutes or until medium-rare.
3. Shake the frying pan continuously to sear the beef cubes uniformly.
4. Position the cooked beef in the slow cooker, then put in the stock cube, mixed herbs, garlic, onions, salt, black pepper, and water.
5. Stir to mix thoroughly.

6. Place the slow cooker lid on and cook on LOW for ten hours.

7. Ladle the stew in a big container and serve warm.

Slow Cooker Lamb & Cauliflower Soup

Time To Prepare: ten minutes
Time to Cook: 4 hours
Yield: Servings 6

Ingredients:

- ½ teaspoon cracked black pepper
- ½ teaspoon salt
- 1 cauliflower head, cut into florets
- 1 cup heavy cream
- 1 pound ground lamb
- 1 tablespoon freshly chopped thyme
- 1 yellow onion, chopped
- 2 cloves garlic, chopped
- 5 cups beef broth

Directions:

1. Put in the ground lamb and cauliflower to the base of a stockpot.

2. Put in the rest of the ingredients minus the heavy cream, and cook on high for 4 hours.

3. Warm the heavy cream before you put it in the soup.

4. Use an immersion blender to combine the soup until creamy.

Sugars Spicy Cabbage Turmeric Coconut Soup

TimeTo Prepare: ten minutes
Time to Cook: twenty minutes
Yield: Servings 4

Ingredients:

- ½ teaspoon black pepper
- ½ teaspoon salt
- 1 head white cabbage
- 1 teaspoon cumin powder
- 1/4 cup coconut milk
- 2 cloves garlic
- 2 tablespoons coconut oil
- 2 teaspoons turmeric powder
- 3 cups vegetable/chicken stock

Directions:

1. Heat the oil in a frying pan on moderate heat.
2. Put in the cabbage & garlic & sauté until the cabbage is delicate.
3. Put in the stock, bubble, spread, & stew for about twenty minutes.
4. Turn off the heat, including the coconut milk & flavors.
5. Blend until the desired smoothness is achieved & season to taste.
6. Serve, gulp & appreciate!

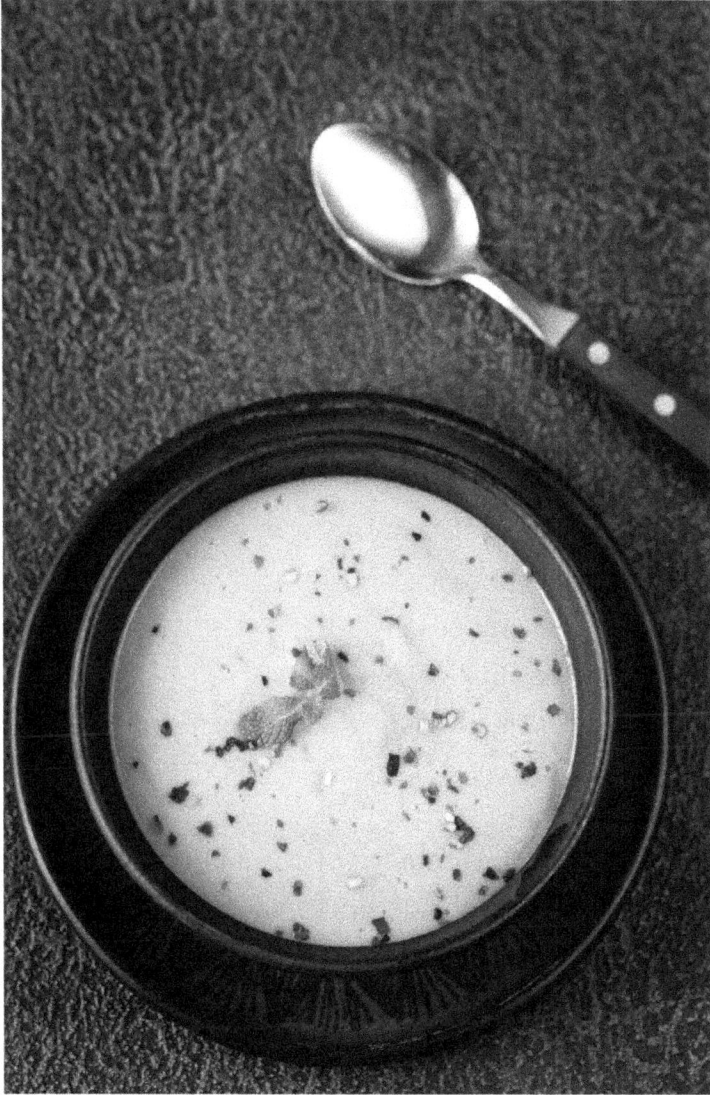

Spicy Ramen Noodles

Time To Prepare: fifteen minutes
Time to Cook: 0 minutes
Yield: Servings 4

Ingredients:
- ¼ cup chopped fresh cilantro
- ¼ cup cut scallion
- ¼ cup thinly cut cucumber
- 1 tablespoon coconut aminos
- 1 tablespoon freshly squeezed lime juice
- 1 tablespoon grated peeled fresh ginger
- 1 tablespoon raw honey
- 1 teaspoon chili powder
- 2 tablespoons rice vinegar
- 2 tablespoons sesame oil
- 2 tablespoons sesame seeds
- 8 ounces buckwheat noodles or rice noodles, cooked

Directions:
1. In a big serving container, meticulously mix the noodles, sesame seeds, cucumber, scallion, cilantro, sesame oil, vinegar, ginger, coconut aminos, honey, lime juice, and chili powder.
2. Split among 4 soup bowls and serve at room temperature

Sweet Potato and Black Bean Chili

Time To Prepare: ten minutes
Time to Cook: twenty minutes
Yield: Servings 8

Ingredients:
- ¼ teaspoon cayenne pepper
- ¼ teaspoon dried oregano
- ½ teaspoon ground cinnamon
- 1 (28-ounce) can diced tomatoes with their juice
- 1 green bell pepper, diced
- 1 red bell pepper, diced
- 1 red onion, diced
- 1 tablespoon chili powder
- 1 tablespoon freshly squeezed lime juice
- 1 teaspoon cocoa powder
- 1 teaspoon ground cumin
- 1 teaspoon salt
- 2 cups vegetable broth
- 2 tablespoons avocado oil
- 3 cups black beans, drained and washed well
- 3 cups cooked sweet potato cubes
- 5 garlic cloves, minced

Directions:
1. In a huge soup pot on moderate heat, warm the avocado oil.
2. Place the onion and garlic, and sauté for a couple of minutes.
3. Mix in the red bell pepper and the green bell pepper, and sauté for approximately 3 minutes until tender.

4. Put in the sweet potato, beans, broth, tomatoes, lime juice, chili powder, cocoa powder, cumin, salt, cinnamon, cayenne pepper, and oregano, then stir until blended.
5. Put to a simmer, and cook for fifteen minutes.
6. Serve instantly

Tex-Mex Chicken Soup

Time To Prepare: ten minutes
Time to Cook: 1 hour
Yield: Servings 4

Ingredients:

- ¼ cup roasted pumpkin seeds
- 1 teaspoon paprika powder
- 1 yellow onion, chopped
- 1¾ cups coconut cream
- 12 ounces (340 g) boneless chicken thighs
- 2 tablespoons coconut oil
- 3 tablespoons Tex-Mex seasoning
- 4 tablespoons lime juice
- Fresh cilantro, chopped
- Salt and ground black pepper, to taste

Directions:

1. Cook the chicken thighs in a pot of water, covered, for thirty minutes or until the chicken is completely fork-soft.

2. Move the chicken to a container and reserve the chicken broth until ready to use.

3. Warm the coconut oil in a nonstick frying pan on moderate heat, then put in the onion and drizzle with Tex-Mex seasoning, salt, and pepper. sauté for five minutes until the onion is translucent.

4. Pour over the reserved chicken broth and coconut cream.

5. Bring them to a simmer for about twenty minutes or until it becomes thick.

6. Put in the chicken, pumpkin seeds, paprika powder, lime juice, and cilantro to the soup.

7. Stir to blend well before you serve.

Creamy Cauliflower Soup

Yield: 4-6 servings
Preparation Time: fifteen minutes
Cooking Time: 22-25 minutes

Ingredients:

- 1 tablespoon extra-virgin extra virgin olive oil
- 1 medium onion, chopped
- 4 garlic cloves, minced
- Salt, to taste
- 1 medium head cauliflower, cut into 1-inch pieces
- 4 ½-5½ cups water
- 1 avocado, peeled, pitted and chopped
- 2-3 cups mixed greens
- Freshly ground black pepper, to taste
- Fresh chopped parsley, for garnishing

Directions:

1. In a substantial soup pan, heat oil on medium heat.

2. Add onion and sauté for approximately 4-5 minutes.

3. Add garlic and pinch of salt and sauté approximately 2-3 minutes.

4. Stir in cauliflower and add water. Bring with a boil on high heat.

5. Reduce the heat to low. Simmer for about 10 minutes.

6. Stir in avocado and greens and simmer for about 3 minutes.

7. Remove from heat and cool slightly.

8. In a blender, transfer the soup in batches and pulse till smooth.

9. Add the soup within the pan on medium heat. Cook for around 3-4 minutes.

10. Stir in salt and black pepper and take off from heat.

11. Serve with all the garnishing of parsley.

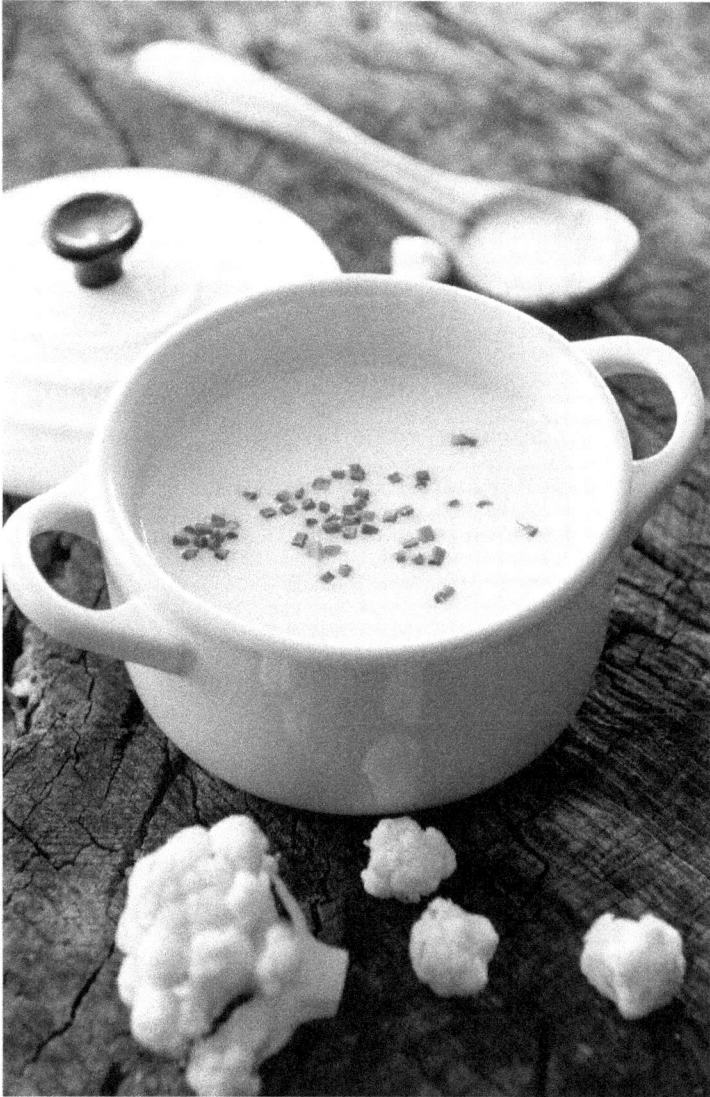

Green Veggie Soup

Yield: 6 servings
Preparation Time: 20 min
Cooking Time: 25 minutes

Ingredients:
- 2 tablespoons ghee (clarified butter)
- 3-4 garlic cloves, minced
- 4 leeks (white part), chopped roughly
- 2 medium heads broccoli, chopped roughly
- ½ of small head cauliflower, chopped roughly
- 4 celery sticks, chopped roughly
- 8 cups homemade vegetable broth
- 2-3 cups fresh baby spinach
- 1 cup fresh parsley, chopped
- Freshly ground black pepper, to taste
- Pinch of ground nutmeg
- 1 tablespoon coconut cream

Directions:
1. In a big soup pan, heat oil on medium heat.
2. Add garlic and leeks and sauté for approximately 4-5 minutes.
3. Add broccoli, cauliflower and celery and sauté for approximately 5 minutes.
4. Add broth and convey with a boil. Reduce heat to low. Simmer for approximately 10-fifteen minutes.
5. Stir in spinach and parsley and remove from heat.
6. With an immense blender, blend till pureed. Stir in nutmeg and black pepper.
7. Top using the dollop of coconut cream and serve.

Mushroom Soup

Yield: 4 servings
Preparation Time: twenty minutes
Cooking Time: half an hour

Ingredients:

- ½-ounce dried porcini mushrooms
- 2 tablespoons ghee (clarified butter)
- 1 celery stalk, chopped
- 1 large leek (pale part), chopped
- 1 small sweet potato, peeled and chopped
- 15 medium crimini mushrooms, sliced roughly
- 3 garlic cloves, minced
- 1 tablespoon dried thyme, crushed
- 3 cups homemade chicken broth
- ½ teaspoon Dijon mustard
- 1 tablespoon red boat fish sauce
- 2 bay leaves
- 1 teaspoon fresh lemon zest, grated finely
- ½ teaspoon freshly ground black pepper
- 3 tablespoons almond butter
- 1 tablespoon fresh lemon juice

Directions:

1. In a bowl, soak porcini mushrooms in boiling water. Keep aside for about 15- twenty or so minutes.

2. Strain the mushrooms, reserving ½ cup of liquid. Then chop the mushrooms.

3. In a sizable soup pan, heat ghee on medium heat.

4. Add celery and leek and sauté for about 5-7 minutes.

5. Add sweet potato, cremini mushrooms, garlic and thyme and sauté for approximately 1-2 minutes.

6. Add broth, mustard, fish sauce, bay leaves, lemon zest, black pepper and cremini mushrooms with reserved liquid and convey to a boil.

7. Reduce the temperature to low. Cover and simmer for about quarter-hour.

8. Uncover and simmer for 5 minutes more.

9. Stir in almond butter and lemon juice and serve hot.

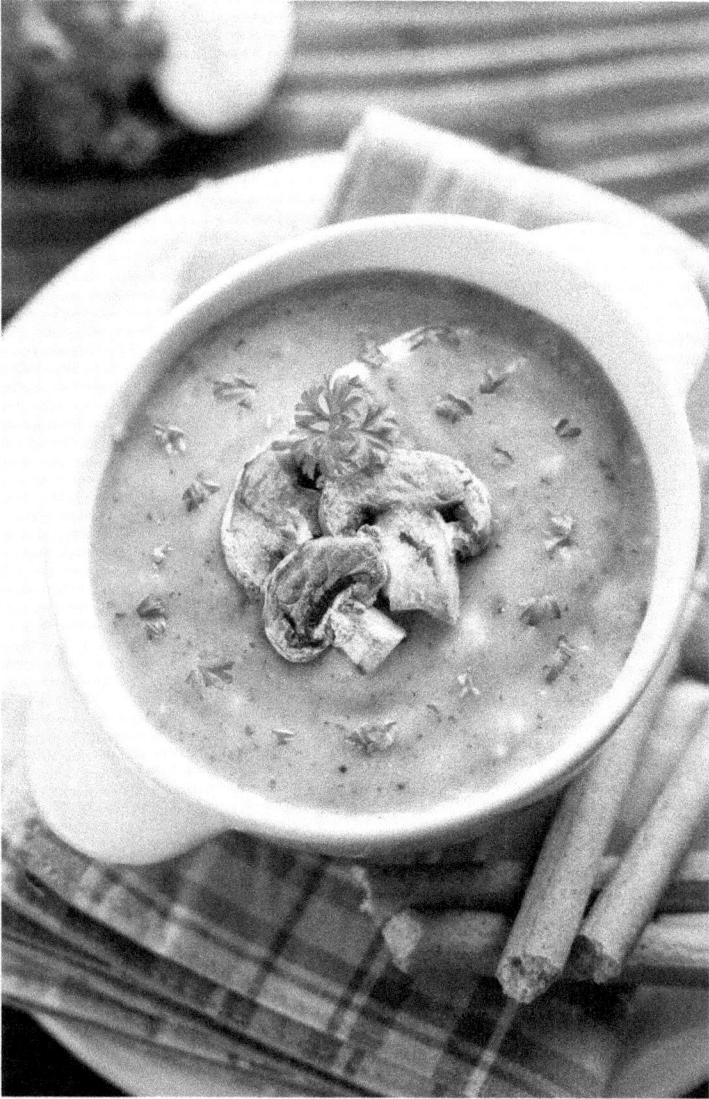

Chicken & Asparagus Soup

Yield: 8 servings
Preparation Time: 20 min
Cooking Time: 20 min

Ingredients:

- 1 tablespoon coconut oil
- 1 onion, chopped
- 2 cups mushrooms, sliced thinly
- 1 celery stalk, chopped
- 2 cups grass-fed boneless chicken, chopped
- 15-20 fresh asparagus spears, trimmed and chopped
- 6-8 cups homemade chicken broth
- 14-ounce coconut milk
- 2 cups fresh spinach, chopped
- Salt and freshly ground black pepper, to taste

Directions:

1. In a big soup pan, heat oil on medium heat.
2. Add onion, mushrooms and celery and sauté for approximately 5 minutes.
3. Add chicken, asparagus and broth and bring to a boil.
4. Reduce heat to low. Simmer for around 10 min.
5. Stir in coconut milk and spinach and bring to your boil on high heat.
6. Reduce the temperature to low. Simmer for around 3-4 minutes.
7. Stir in salt and black pepper and take off from heat.
8. Serve hot.

Zucchini & Squash Soup

Yield: 4 servings
Preparation Time: quarter-hour
Cooking Time: 12-quarter-hour

Ingredients:
- 2 tablespoons coconut oil
- 1 small onion, chopped
- 3 garlic cloves, minced
- 1 teaspoon ground cumin
- 1½ pounds yellow squash, chopped
- 3 cups zucchini, chopped
- 2 tablespoons jalapeño peppers, chopped finely
- 4 cups homemade vegetable broth
- 1 cup coconut milk
- 3 tablespoons fresh lemon juice
- ¼ cup fresh cilantro, chopped
- 2 tablespoons nutritional yeast
- Avocado slices, for garnishing

Directions:
1. In a large soup pan, heat oil on medium heat.
2. Add onion and sauté approximately 4-5 minutes.
3. Add garlic and cumin and sauté approximately 1 minute.
4. Add squash and zucchini and sauté for about 3-4 minutes.
5. Add jalapeño peppers and broth and convey to your boil. Immediately, turn off heat.
6. Keep covered approximately 10 minutes.
7. Stir in coconut milk, fresh lemon juice, cilantro and nutritional yeast and again bring with a boil.
8. Serve hot while using topping of avocado slices.

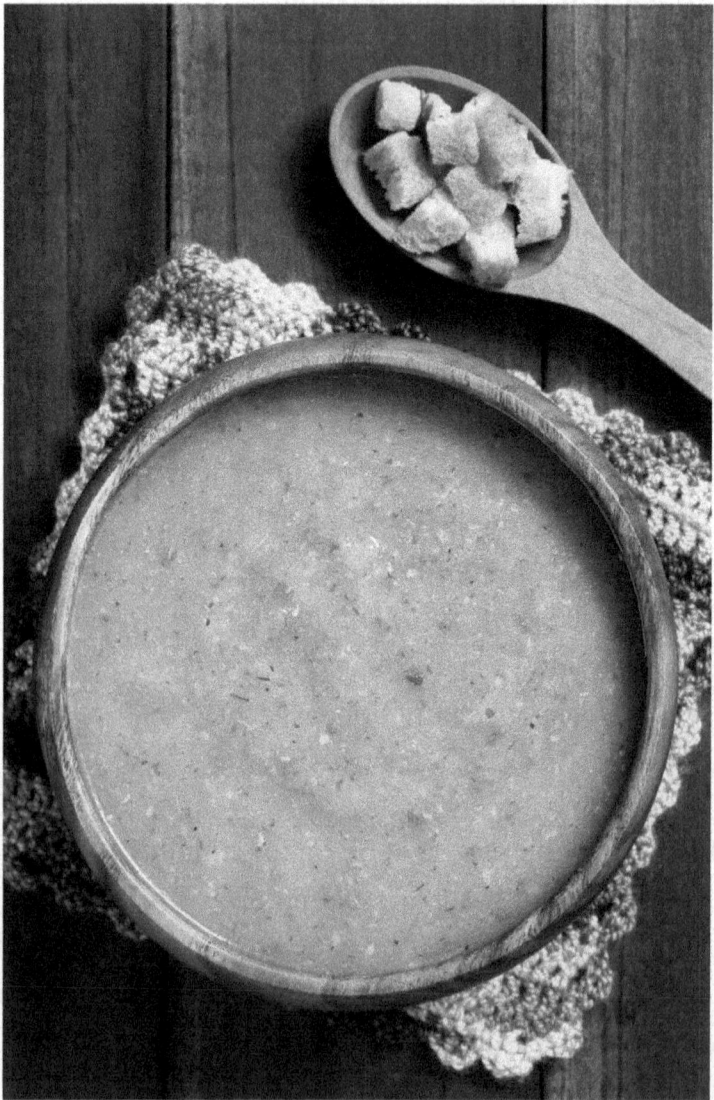

Tuscan Style Soup

Time To Prepare: three minutes
Time to Cook: five minutes
Yield: Servings 4

Ingredients:
- ½ cup leeks, cut
- 1 carrot, trimmed and grated
- 1 zucchini, shredded
- 1/4 teaspoon ground black pepper
- 2 cups broth, if possible homemade
- 2 cups water
- 2 garlic cloves, minced
- 2 tablespoons butter, melted
- 4 cups broccoli rabe, broken into pieces
- Sea salt, to taste

Directions:
1. Push the "Sauté" button to heat up your Instant Pot; now, melt the butter.
2. Cook the leeks for approximately 2 minutes or until tender.
3. Put in minced garlic and cook for an additional 40 seconds.
4. Put in the rest of the ingredients.
5. Secure the lid. "Manual" mode and Low pressure; cook for about three minutes.
6. Once cooking is complete, use a quick pressure release; cautiously remove the lid.
7. Enjoy

Vegetarian Garlic, Tomato & Onion Soup

Time To Prepare: fifteen minutes
Time to Cook: thirty minutes
Yield: Servings 6

Ingredients:
- ½ cup full-fat unsweetened coconut milk
- 1 bay leaf
- 1 teaspoon Italian seasoning
- 1 yellow onion, chopped
- 1½ cups canned diced tomatoes
- 3 cloves garlic, chopped
- 6 cups vegetable broth
- Fresh basil, for serving
- Pinch of salt & pepper, to taste

Directions:
1. Put in all the ingredients minus the coconut milk and fresh basil to a stockpot on moderate heat and bring to its boiling point.
2. Reduce to a simmer and cook for half an hour
3. Take away the bay leaf, and then use an immersion blender to combine the soup until the desired smoothness is achieved.
4. Mix in the coconut milk.
5. Decorate using fresh basil before you serve.

White Velvet Cauliflower Soup

Time ToPrepare: ten minutes
Time to Cook: twenty minutes
Yield: Servings 6

Ingredients:
- 1 head cauliflower, chopped into 1-inch pieces
- 1 small celery root, peeled, cut into 1-inch pieces
- 1 small white onion, diced
- 1 tbsp. avocado oil
- 2 scallions, cut
- 2 tbsp. ghee
- 3 garlic cloves, minced
- 4 cups vegetable broth

Directions:
1. In a huge soup pot on moderate heat, heat the avocado oil.
2. Place the onion and garlic, and sauté for five minutes.
3. Place the celery root and cauliflower.
4. Raise the heat to moderate-high, then continue to sauté for minimum five minutes, or until the cauliflower starts to brown and caramelize the sides.
5. Mix in the broth and ghee and place it to its boiling point.
6. Lessen the heat to moderate-low and simmer for about ten minutes.
7. Take away the pot from the heat.
8. Use an immersion blender to or in batches in a standard blender, purée the soup until creamy.
9. Serve instantly, sprinkled with the scallions.

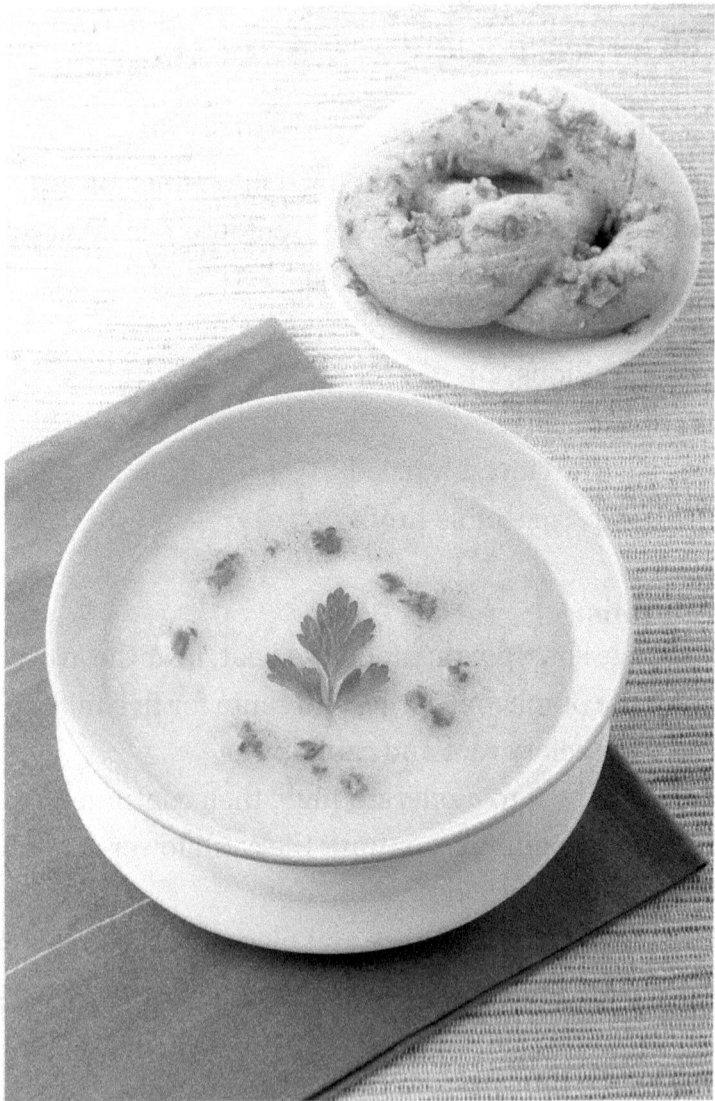

106

Sugars Zesty Broccoli Soup

TimeTo Prepare: ten minutes
Time to Cook: twenty minutes
Yield: Servings 4

Ingredients:

- ½ teaspoon freshly squeezed lemon juice
- ½ teaspoon lemon zest
- ½ teaspoon salt
- 1 carrot, chopped
- 1 celery stalk, diced
- 1 head broccoli, roughly chopped
- 1 medium white onion, diced
- 1 tablespoon ghee
- 3 cups vegetable broth
- 3 garlic cloves, minced
- Freshly ground black pepper

Directions:

1.In a huge soup pot on moderate heat, melt the ghee.

2. Place the onion and garlic, and sauté for five minutes.

3. Put in the broccoli, carrot, and celery, and sauté for a couple of minutes.

4. Mix in the broth, salt, lemon juice, and lemon zest, and flavor with pepper.

5. Heat to a simmer, and cook for minimum ten minutes.

6. Serve instantly.

Carrot Soup

Yield: 8 servings
Preparation Time: fifteen minutes
Cooking Time: 1 hour 40 minutes

Ingredients:
- 2 pounds carrots, peeled and cut into slices
- 7 tablespoons extra-virgin essential olive oil, divided
- 2 large fennel bulbs, sliced
- Salt, to taste
- ¼ cup pumpkin seeds
- 1 medium yellow onion, chopped
- 6 garlic cloves, minced
- 1 tablespoon fresh ginger, grated
- 1 tablespoon ground turmeric
- ½ teaspoon red pepper cayenne
- 2 tablespoons fresh lime juice
- 1½ cups coconut milk
- 4-6 cups water
- ¼ cup scallion (green part), minced

Directions:
1. Preheat the oven to 375 degrees F.
2. In a baking sheet, place the carrot and drizzle with 2 tablespoons of oil.
3. Roast approximately one hour.
4. Remove the carrots from oven and set aside.
5. Now, raise the temperature of oven to 400 degrees F.
6. In a skillet, heat 3 tablespoons of oil on medium heat.

7. Add fennel bulbs and pinch of salt and sauté for about 4-5 minutes.

8. Transfer the fennel bulb onto a baking sheet and roast approximately 20-a half-hour.

9. Meanwhile, heat a nonstick skillet on medium heat. Keep aside.

10. Add pumpkin seeds and stir fry for around 3-4 minutes or till toasted. Keep aside.

11. Meanwhile in a very soup pan, heat remaining oil on medium heat.

12. Add onion and sauté for around 12 minutes.

13. Add garlic and sauté for approximately 1 minute.

14. In a blender, add onion mixture, carrots, ginger, spices, lime juice and coconut milk and pulse till well combined.

15. Add required amount of water and pulse till smooth.

16. Return the soup in the pan on medium heat.

17. Bring to some boil and cook for approximately 3-5 minutes.

18. Serve hot with all the topping of fennel and pumpkin seeds.

Notes

www.ingramcontent.com/pod-product-compliance
Lightning Source LLC
Chambersburg PA
CBHW050800030426
42336CB00012B/1882